STATE *of* SLIM

Fix Your **Metabolism** and Drop
20 Pounds in 8 Weeks on the **Colorado Diet**

James O. Hill, PhD, AND Holly R. Wyatt, MD
with Christie Aschwanden

RODALE.

© 2013 by James O. Hill, PhD, and Holly R. Wyatt, MD

Rodale books may be purchased for business or promotional use or for special sales. For information, please write to:
Special Markets Department, Rodale Inc., 733 Third Avenue, New York, NY 10017.

Printed in the United States of America
Rodale Inc. makes every effort to use acid-free ♾, recycled paper ♻.

Book design by Kara Plikaitis

Library of Congress Cataloging-in-Publication Data is on file with the publisher
ISBN-13: 978–1–60961–491–1 hardcover

Distributed to the trade by Macmillan
2 4 6 8 10 9 7 5 3 1 hardcover

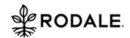

We inspire and enable people to improve their lives and the world around them.
rodalebooks.com

For my wife, Trish, and my sons, Alex and Michael
—JOH

For my father, Charles Larry Thompson
—HRW

CONTENTS

ACKNOWLEDGMENTS

WE WANT TO GIVE special thanks to our colleague Dr. John Peters. John has been our collaborator for many years. He provided insight, advice, and critique on every chapter in this book. We are very happy he has joined our research group at the University of Colorado.

We are so grateful to our patients, our research participants, our fellow Coloradans, and the members of the National Weight Control Registry. We wrote this book to share what we have learned from them. They continue to inspire us to keep learning and to get better at helping people manage their weight.

We have published several research papers describing what we have learned from the National Weight Control Registry. All of this research has been conducted in collaboration with Dr. Rena Wing and her colleagues at Brown University. Rena has been a wonderful friend and colleague for many years and is one of the best researchers in our field.

We have had the opportunity to work and collaborate with many brilliant obesity scientists, and we've learned so much from them. We want to thank the National Institutes of Health (NIH) for funding our research over the past years. Our approach to weight management is science-based, and most of the science of weight regulation was developed with NIH support.

We have received unwavering support from our collaborators and colleagues at the University of Colorado (CU). The CU leadership team, especially Bruce and Marcy Benson, Lilly Marks, Dick Krugman, and Chip Ridgway, have supported and encouraged us to make CU the best place in the world for obesity research. We want to thank our coworkers at the Anschutz Health and Wellness Center who work tirelessly on our research studies and in our wellness clinic. We want to give special thanks to Phillip Anschutz who helped make the Anschutz Health and Wellness Center a reality and a place where people can enroll in state-of-the-art programs for weight management, including the Colorado Diet. He not only believes in wellness, he walks the talk.

A project like this one takes a team and we have a good one. We were fortunate to work with Trisha Calvo at Rodale. She had a vision for this book from the beginning. She is both talented and patient, and the book is much better because of her editing. James Levine, our agent, worked long and hard to make this happen and has provided sound advice to us all along. Christie Aschwanden worked beside us every step of the way. Her skills both in writing and in nutrition helped make the science and the advice more understandable and relevant.

Finally, we are both grateful that we found our way to Colorado and have the opportunity to live the Colorado lifestyle.

From Jim:

Thank you to my wife, Trish, and my sons, Alex and Michael, for your support, encouragement, and understanding of my long hours and many days away from home. And thanks, Alex, for letting me share your story on page 55.

From Holly:

Thank you to my parents. My dad instilled my love for science and taught me how to think critically and to ask questions about everything. He is my role model for working hard and living with integrity. Even after his death, he has continued to guide me and show me the importance of following my purpose. I am so grateful and I know I will see him again one day.

And my mother has always been my biggest supporter. She says that raising her "girls" was the best job she could ever have. I would not have gotten through medical school without her sacrifice and support. You are the best, Mom, period!

INTRODUCTION

As WEIGHT-LOSS RESEARCHERS WHO'VE published hundreds of scientific papers and helped thousands of people lose weight, we've seen diet trends come and go—some of them more than once! Frankly, diets don't work (that's why there are so many of them). So why, then, are we writing a diet book?

Well, *State of Slim* isn't *really* a diet book. Yes, we give you a step-by-step plan for eating and exercising the healthiest way. And yes, you'll lose weight—quickly and safely. But we think you deserve more.

Typical diet books contain quick-fix plans designed to help you fit into your skinny jeans or look thinner for a one-night class reunion. They lure you with promises of dramatic results (drop 15 pounds in 15 days!). And it's true, you can lose weight with any one of these plans—but you probably won't keep it off. Even though you're trying to do all the right things, the pounds inevitably will creep back on, and you won't have a clue how to stop them. You'll probably assume that the weight regain is your fault, feel terrible, and repeat the whole sad process with the next new diet book.

You deserve to know the real deal: Dropping pounds is only

part of the picture. You aren't overweight simply because you eat too much and therefore must "diet" to slim down. Lack of movement has played an important role as well. In fact, overeating is just as much a *consequence* of being overweight as it is a cause (we'll explain this startling fact later on). Keeping weight off is a different challenge than losing weight and requires a different strategy. Our approach, which we call the Colorado Diet, tackles both aspects. It is a complete and permanent solution to your weight problem.

———

By now you must be wondering why we call the *State of Slim* plan the Colorado Diet. We both live in the Denver area, and we run the Anschutz Health and Wellness Center at the University of Colorado. But that's not the only reason. At a time when two-thirds of the American population is overweight or obese, Colorado has bucked the trend: It's the leanest state in the nation. Colorado has an overall obesity rate of 21 percent, and some counties have obesity rates below 15 percent. Compare this with the national average obesity rate of 28 percent, and 35 percent in the heaviest state. How do those statistics help you if you live in New York, Texas, or Iowa? Our Rocky Mountain state is beautiful and inspiring, but it's not magical. Colorado just happens to provide an opportune place and supportive environment for people to live a lean lifestyle naturally. And our work with our patients—as well as our research with people from all 50 states—has shown that you can adopt a Colorado lifestyle no matter where you live.

Neither one of us is originally from Colorado. When our careers brought us here and we each settled into the Rocky Mountain lifestyle, we found ourselves skiing, hiking, biking, working out, and eating a healthy diet—like many of our colleagues, neighbors, and friends—and feeling healthier. (Holly's story on page xvi will likely resonate with many of you.) At the same time, we were both involved in a research project that Jim cofounded. Called the National Weight Control Registry (NWCR), it's a scientific database of more than 10,000 people from across the country who have dropped at least 30 pounds and maintained the loss for a minimum of a year. The average NWCR participant has lost 70 pounds and kept them off for 6 years. By studying this group, we've identified some key strategies that are essential to successful weight loss and maintenance. And as we learned more about what keeps people lean, we realized that our friends, neighbors, and families were intuitively following those key strategies. That's when it dawned on us: Colorado is the sweet spot where research lab meets real life.

As scientists, we performed many research studies to examine metabolism and obesity. And the top complaint of patients in our weight-loss clinic is "My metabolism isn't working!" When we first began our research, though, we didn't find anything wrong with the metabolisms of overweight and obese people; their bodies burned calories at the exact rate they should. But eventually, we discovered that our patients were right. Overweight people burn calories at a normal rate, but their metabolisms are stuck in a fat-storing mode. We'll explain this more in Chapter 2. For now, know this: You can lose weight with a broken metabolism, but you cannot keep it off.

A Colorado lifestyle creates what we call a Mile-High Metabolism. Denver is known as the Mile-High City because it sits at an elevation of 5,280 feet—exactly a mile above sea level. And with our plan, your metabolism will reach new heights.

Coloradans' lifestyles keep their metabolisms in tip-top

(continued on page xix)

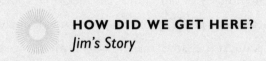

HOW DID WE GET HERE?
Jim's Story

I spent my childhood in a small town in Tennessee before going off
to college and then graduate school. I've been studying obesity and
weight loss since 1981. The first research I ever published showed
that if you give rats a high-fat diet, they get fatter than if you feed
them a low-fat diet. The same study also revealed that rats who
exercise don't get as fat as the other rats, even if they gobble fatty
food. I wanted to know if the same things happened in humans
(they do), so in the late 1980s I began conducting weight-loss studies with people. In my research, I have found that there are many
ways to lose weight but that most people who lose it are not able
to keep it off. It seemed to me that for a weight-loss program to be
effective, it has to work for both losing weight *and* keeping it off.

One evening in 1993, while attending a research conference, I
went out for a drink with Dr. Rena Wing, a psychologist now at
Brown University and one of the leading weight-loss researchers in
the world. As we sat at the bar and nursed our drinks, our conversation turned to a curious fact. The media at the time made it sound as
if no one ever managed to lose weight and keep it off. Scientists
were so busy studying the people who failed that no one had both-
ered to look at the people who were succeeding, to figure out how
they did it. It was a eureka moment. We looked at each other and
realized that we'd stumbled upon something *big*. We decided then
and there that we would find people who'd successfully slimmed

down and discover their strategies and secrets. That evening, the National Weight Control Registry (NWCR) was born.

In the 18 years since we launched it, the NWCR has become a primary source of information about how successful weight-loss maintainers behave. We now have more than 10,000 people in the registry, all of whom have kept off at least 30 pounds for a minimum of 1 year. The average person in the NWCR has lost around 70 pounds and kept it off for about 6 years. These stories of triumph have taught us important, and sometimes surprising, lessons about what it takes to succeed.

In 1992, I moved to the University of Colorado to develop the world's premier research group studying nutrition, weight management, and physical activity. Our group has conducted many research studies aimed at better understanding how to lose weight and keep it off. We knew that Colorado is America's leanest state, but it's only in recent years that Holly Wyatt and I realized that a few crucial lifestyle factors explain why and how so many Coloradans stay slender. This was my second big eureka moment. I recognized these key factors right away, because I'd seen them before. What now seems obvious came as an epiphany—participants in the NWCR live like Coloradans. And that's exciting, because people in the NWCR live all over the country. Colorado made lean living famous, but participants in the NWCR prove that you can adopt the Colorado lifestyle *anywhere*.

HOW DID WE GET HERE?
Holly's Story

Growing up in Houston, I was always a little thicker (okay, fatter) than the other kids. I was an A student but lacked even an ounce of natural athletic talent. I hated PE class. The annual Presidential Physical Fitness Test reduced me to tears every time. For the life of me, I could not master the bar hang. I never passed the test. Despite my lack of natural ability, I tried out for the drill team during my freshman year of high school. I struggled to learn the dance moves, but I made the team. Then came the dreaded weekly weigh-ins. Every Friday, I was required to step on the scale. If the number read 133 or less, I was allowed on the field to perform with the team. If the scale hit 134, I was relegated to the sidelines. I started fixating on my weight and wondering why the other girls on the dance squad could eat so much more pizza and candy than I could without worrying about weigh-in time.

During my premed studies at the University of Texas, I stopped dancing and gained the fabled "freshman 15." My weight continued to climb over the next 4 years. When I got to medical school at Baylor College of Medicine in Houston, I started experimenting with different diets. The demanding hours of residency left me no time for exercise, and my weight proceeded to fluctuate up and down. With each new diet, the outcome was the same: I'd lose weight, but it always came back.

I continued bouncing from one diet to the next during my residency in internal medicine at the University of Colorado. One day, my attending physician spied me eating four hard-boiled eggs after my rounds. He asked me what I was doing, and I explained that I was on one of the high-protein diets popular at the time. He told me I was going to rot my kidneys and suggested I talk to an endocrinologist who studied obesity. His advice that day began a cascade of events that changed my career path. We didn't learn about obesity in medical school, and until then, I'd never realized that metabolism and obesity were things I could specialize in and study scientifically.

Against the advice of some of my advisors (who insisted I needed to study under a physician, not a PhD scientist), I selected Dr. Jim Hill as my research mentor. Jim had recently started the NWCR, and I recognized immediately that the registry would provide the perfect resource for testing ideas and strategies for weight loss. Jim shared everything he knew and taught me the nuts and bolts of how to do research. That was more than 15 years ago, and we've been collaborators ever since.

Jim has shaped my thinking on weight loss, but some of my most important insights have come from my patients and my own experiences as a serial dieter. Early in my practice, I noted that many people who came to my obesity clinic insisted that something was wrong with their metabolisms—they couldn't eat the same things their spouse or sister or best friend could without gaining weight. Initially, I dismissed their stories. The

(continued)

Holly's Story—Continued

science at that time didn't offer any evidence to back up the idea that their metabolisms were faulty. In fact, one of the first studies I did with Jim showed that people in the NWCR had perfectly normal metabolisms. But our research since then has proved those frustrated dieters correct. Our obese patients *do* have metabolisms that are stuck in a fat-storage mode, and losing weight alone won't fix them. Because metabolism drops along with the pounds, people who have been obese have to work much harder than normal-weight people to prevent weight gain. That's the discouraging news, but we've found good news, too. The fact that people in the NWCR had normal metabolisms wasn't proof that their metabolisms were never broken; instead, it was evidence that these successful dieters had managed to fix the problems that obesity had inflicted on their metabolisms. Our research has not only proved that it's possible to repair a broken metabolism, but it showed us how. I'm one of the "easy gainers" we describe in Chapter 2, but the science I've learned working with Jim showed me how to end my weight woes for good. Now we're sharing what we have learned with you.

shape—revved up and able to easily burn whatever they eat. It all starts with physical activity. For many Coloradans, it's not a matter of deciding *whether* to exercise—it's choosing what to do, when, and with whom.

When you stop moving your body, your metabolism slows, your appetite goes haywire, and you begin eating too much of the wrong kinds of foods. The result? You gain weight and have difficulty losing those extra pounds. You just can't be healthy and slim without regular physical activity—and we say that with decades of research behind us to prove it. We'll show you how to incorporate an achievable, enjoyable amount of physical activity into your life—in effect, creating your own Colorado lifestyle—so that your body's metabolism works with you to stay at a healthy weight.

Of course, what you eat is also important. Colorado cuisine can be described as fresh, flavorful, and seasonal. We eat smarter, not less. And the foods we choose to eat help keep our metabolisms revved instead of bringing it to a near stop.

In Colorado, when friends get together, they're more likely to meet up for a hike, a bike ride, or a day on the slopes than they are to go out to a restaurant together. Certainly, exercising is easier when everyone you know is doing it and you have lots of options year-round. But it's not just about living in the right location. It's about attitude and approach. No matter where you live, we'll show you how to tweak your physical and social environments and develop healthy routines and rituals so that it becomes easy to create and maintain this lifestyle forever.

———

To help you achieve a Mile-High Metabolism, we first give you an understanding of the skills you need to keep your weight off. Most diets aim to stop bad habits. Ours focuses on instilling good ones. The difference may seem subtle, but our research suggests that it's anything but.

Remember how we said that losing weight requires a different approach than maintaining that loss? While you are losing weight with the Colorado Diet, you will be preparing yourself for long-term success even before you start—something no other plan does for you. There are three phases. Phase 1 will *reignite* your fat burners so you lose weight quickly—typically 8 to 10 pounds. Phase 2 will *rebuild* your metabolism. You'll continue to drop pounds and strengthen your metabolism while your diet variety increases. In phase 3, you'll *reinforce* your metabolism by finding a pattern of physical activity that keeps your Mile-High Metabolism stoked and fueled by a smart, healthy, satisfying diet. You'll now be ready to live the Colorado lifestyle we outline in Chapter 9—forever.

We're tired of watching people succeed in losing weight, only to regain it all within a few months. We're tired of seeing people sentenced to a life of food restriction and deprivation. As scientists and researchers, we haven't just theorized about the right weight-loss strategies, we've tested them in our clinic to see if they really work—and they do. Isn't it time to not just lose weight but fix your metabolism so you can join the ranks of those who have succeeded?

What Makes Colorado Special?

CHAPTER I

WE'RE FREQUENTLY ASKED BY the media and by people we meet at parties why America is getting so fat. Is it because we spend too much time sitting in front of the TV? Is it because we drink those huge sugary soft drinks or that junk food advertising is often geared toward kids? Everyone has an opinion: Healthy food is too expensive. Schools are the problem, since most did away with recess and serve unhealthy food. Our portion sizes are too big, and we're eating too many wheat-based products. The list is endless. People want to blame someone or one specific thing—and everyone wants a simple solution.

There's no doubt that overweight and obesity are huge health problems in our country. Americans have been gaining weight year after year since the early 1980s. In fact, we published a study in *Science* in 2003 showing that the average weight gain in adults is about 2 pounds per year. This may not seem like a lot, but it adds up to 20 extra pounds in a decade!

What has caused this increase in weight gain? The American lifestyle has changed so much in the past 30 years—nearly everything about the places we live, work, and play is different—that it's impossible to assign blame to any one, two, or even three things. More important, though, we don't believe that "Why is America getting so fat?" is the right question. There *are* people who are lean and healthy. Some of them have always been this way; others have managed to lose weight and keep it off for a very long time. We've been asking, "How do these people do it?" With the Colorado Diet, our focus is on what people have done right.

Colorado is a perfect learning laboratory in which to study what's effective and what isn't for weight loss because there are many, many people here doing it right. While the rest of the nation has been packing on the pounds, Coloradans have avoided the high rates of obesity seen elsewhere. The state has the lowest obesity prevalence in the nation, about 26 percent below the national average. However, not everyone in Colorado is lean—just being a Coloradan doesn't give you immunity against the factors that contribute to obesity. You have to live the Colorado lifestyle actively.

In studying the Colorado lifestyle, we discovered six key factors that make healthy living easy and are necessary for developing a Mile-High Metabolism (we describe this in greater detail in Chapter 2). We think they explain why Coloradans are the leanest people in the nation. What's more, in comparing the habits of lean Coloradans to those of the participants in the National Weight Control Registry (NWCR), we determined that you don't need be a Colorado resident to adopt this lifestyle. Those people live across the country, proving you can be a weight-loss success story anywhere. In the chapters that follow, we'll go into greater detail about each one of the factors and show you how to incorporate them into your daily life. But for now, we wanted to give you an overview.

1 / Be Active Every Day

A few years ago, we worked with Harris Polls to research the walking habits of people across the United States and published the results in the journal *Medicine and Science in Sports and Exercise*. Participants wore pedometers to count the number of steps they took each day. Turns out that the national average was about 5,500 steps (about 2 to 2½ miles), but Coloradans took 1,000 additional steps. We weren't surprised to find that obesity rates were correlated to the number of steps taken. In Arkansas and Tennessee, where obesity rates are among the highest in the country, residents took only 4,500 steps per day.

There's no getting around it—to stay lean, you must be consistently active. Without regular movement, your metabolism becomes slow, sluggish, and inflexible. And an inflexible metabolism makes weight gain inevitable and lasting weight loss next to impossible. Whether it's a walk with the dog, a hike with a friend, a bike ride, or a workout at the gym, movement is a priority in Colorado, not another dreaded task on the to-do list. Some of us get up early, others fit it in between obligations, but the key is we always find a way.

If this feels foreign and seems daunting to you now, don't despair. In Chapter 4, we help you discover the joy of movement and show you how to make it part of your life.

2 / Fuel Up on Real Food

With all that activity, Coloradans love to eat, but we're selective about our food. We look for fresh and local fare, sustainably grown and harvested, where possible. Just about every neighborhood has a farmers' market, and health and organic food stores are very popular, too. (In fact, several major health food chains originated in Colorado.) The majority of our calories come from minimally processed foods that deliver the most flavor and nutrition so our bodies perform at their best. We don't waste our calories on foods with low nutritional value, although we do love our occasional indulgences.

A passion for adventure and new experiences is common here, and food is no exception. Many Coloradans identify as "foodies" and love to cook and seek out inventive restaurants that serve fresh, delicious meals. At restaurants and at home, the emphasis is on quality, not quantity. A healthy-size portion of a great-tasting dish is better than a huge serving of fare that's filled with refined carbohydrates, fat, and sodium—even if that big portion costs less money.

Our friends Debbie and Tim exemplify the Colorado Diet philosophy we discuss in Chapter 5. They love to cook, and even though they live in downtown Denver, they grow their own vegetables in the neighborhood community garden. On a typical Sunday, they might walk or bike to the grocery stores in their neighborhood to pick up a few ingredients for dinner. Debbie prefers making simple meals with fresh ingredients. One of their favorite dinners is sautéed vegetables and herbs tossed with pasta and topped with a little Parmesan cheese—it's tasty, and Debbie can put it together in just a few minutes after work. The couple joined a local farm share program that provides them with a box of fresh, locally produced foods each week. They are both lean and active and readily admit that a major reason they are active is to be able to enjoy the food they love.

3 / Create Your Own Healthy Environment

Colorado is famous for its beautiful scenery and ample opportunities for outdoor recreation. Active people are drawn to our state because of our weather (more than 300 days of sunshine a year), mountains, walking and biking trails, and lots of parks and open spaces. It's hard to stay inside. Of course, it's easier to be active when you're in this kind of environment.

But the typical Coloradan doesn't hike a tall peak before breakfast every day—or even once a month. It's our communities and immediate surroundings—the plethora of parks, the bike paths in our neighborhoods, and our friendly walking groups—that provide an important nudge for healthy living.

And if you're looking for someone to join you on a hike or a bike ride, you don't have to look far. In Colorado, you're likely to rub elbows with a triathlete or trail runner or hiker at a movie, party, or neighborhood event. Your neighbor may be the local running club coach or the organizer of a local charity walk. It seems like everyone owns a bike and a dog. It's not uncommon to begin conversations by talking about the last race you walked or ran rather than what you do for a living. These interactions make living an active lifestyle the norm. This "social circle effect" is exemplified by research done at Harvard University that found that people in the same social network (i.e., groups of friends) tended to have similar body mass indices (body mass index is a measure of obesity). If you're surrounded by friends and family who are overweight, you're more likely to be overweight. Now, this doesn't mean that obesity is contagious; rather it's just that you're likely to engage in the same eating and physical activity patterns as the people you spend most of your time with. And it goes both ways—surround yourself with active people and you become more active, too.

4 / Stay True to Your Purpose

We all have an inner purpose (what we want to accomplish with our lives), but you may not have ever connected your purpose with weight-loss success. Consider this: Is the way you are living your life consistent with what you want to achieve? For Coloradans, being in good shape physically gives them the energy and confidence to do the things that are most important to them, whether it's about providing for family, achieving professional success, or pursuing what they've always wanted to do in retirement. If you recognize how losing weight and keeping it off will help you better reach your goals in life, you will have a powerful motivator to succeed. Making that connection is what spurs you to get up early to hit the gym—even if it's icy cold outside—or gives you the willpower to pass on the second portion at dinner. Living healthfully then becomes a key value in your life and provides motivation for everything you do—and that makes it much more likely that you will enjoy the Colorado lifestyle. Finding your purpose and connecting it to your weight loss goals is an essential factor for success. It's part of the Colorado mind-set we discuss in Chapter 3.

5 / Believe You Can Succeed

During your weight-loss journey, you will face many challenges and small setbacks. Dealing with them in a way that doesn't derail your plan requires keeping a positive mind-set. Your mental outlook can determine how effective you are in making permanent changes in your life. If you believe you can't do something, you probably won't. For you to succeed in losing weight and keeping it off, you have to have faith in your power to change and not get caught up in thinking you're a victim and have no control over the things you perceive as barriers to success. It sounds simplistic, but the idea that having a positive attitude can help you achieve amazing results is backed by science. Research psychologist Barbara Fredrickson, PhD, at the University of North Carolina at Chapel Hill, a leader in the field of positive psychology, has shown that cultivating a positive mind-set can enhance relationships, improve work performance, reduce depression, and contribute to better health. In general, Coloradans have an upbeat attitude. It's not that everyone is running around happy all the time. It's more a sensibility that you are responsible for your own happiness. Instead of saying, "I'll believe it when I see it," Coloradans tend to have the mind-set that if you believe it, you will see it. (Chapter 3 discusses this concept in greater detail.)

It's our experience that people who choose to see a lifestyle change in positive terms do much better than those who don't. Consider Melissa, who came to our weight-loss clinic with a negative mind-set. She was constantly talking about all the foods she couldn't eat on her diet plan. She bemoaned the absence of a chocolate doughnut every morning and complained that Sunday football was just not the same without chicken wings, pizza, and her favorite cold beer. She *had* to exercise every day, and that meant getting up earlier—and she hated getting up earlier. She was losing weight but struggling and even told us we were making her life miserable. You could feel the negative energy when you were in the room with her.

To turn things around, we made it a priority to get her to

PARACHUTING INTO WELLNESS

In September 2011, our colleague John Peters, PhD, moved to Denver from Cincinnati to join our group at the Anschutz Health and Wellness Center. He didn't come here seeking to lose weight. Instead, it happened accidentally. We'll let him explain.

I'd visited Colorado many times over the years and always felt drawn to its natural beauty—the Rocky Mountains, the intense sunlight, and the infinite blue sky. When I decided to move here from Ohio, I felt as if I'd literally parachuted into wellness.

One of the first things I noticed in Colorado was the bicycles—they were everywhere! I've always been a cyclist, but until I relocated to Denver, I had to put my bike on the car roof and drive somewhere to ride. Now, in my neighborhood, I'm only a half mile from the High Line Canal bike trail. I hop on my bike at home and ride to the trailhead. There I can connect to a large network of trails that can take me practically anywhere I want to go!

When I first moved in, I assumed my neighborhood was some sort of planned fitness community. People were out walking at all times of the day and night. But eventually, I realized that all this

concentrate on what she liked about her new lifestyle. Each time we met, we asked her to tell us two things she really enjoyed that week and two things she was grateful for. Over time, her mind-set shifted from feeling like a victim to feeling empowered by her ability to create a new way of living. She began to appreciate the walking is perfectly normal in Colorado—whether there's a foot of snow on the ground or it is 100 degrees outside, people are outside doing something active. A park across the street from my home has a 2-mile-long trail around it. The first month that I moved in, I signed up for a 5-K in my neighborhood park in hopes of meeting some new people. In a single weekend, I made connections with an entire group of people I could meet up with for outdoor activities.

My eating habits changed, too. My neighborhood has a farmers' market about 2 blocks away and a natural food store a few miles away, and both of them are on my Saturday grocery route. Surrounded by healthy food, it was much easier to eat well, no willpower required.

Before I knew it, I'd dropped 20 pounds without even trying. And it was all due to the new lifestyle I'd adopted accidentally as my surroundings reshaped my habits. I hadn't gone on a diet, but my weight dipped to exactly what it was when I got married 35 years ago! Thank goodness I gave away the bell bottoms I had back then, otherwise I'd be tempted to wear them. My only regret is that I didn't do this sooner—there's nothing I'm doing now that I couldn't have done back in Ohio.

opportunities and not chafe against the requirements of her new lifestyle. Melissa not only lost 40 pounds but has kept them off for over a year. We even overheard her telling a new patient that you have the power to make this a great experience or a terrible one—it's your choice.

6 / Make Healthy Living Fun

If you're looking for the Colorado secret, this is it. Coloradans don't eat well and live an active lifestyle to stay lean or even to boost their health; they do it because it's pleasurable. Over the years, we've asked hundreds of Coloradans why physical activity and healthy eating are important to them, and their answers are always the same. They enjoy living this way.

This is where the Colorado Diet departs from most diet plans. Our program isn't about deprivation. Other diets instruct you on ways to live on less food, but the Colorado Diet takes a different approach. We want you to feed your body wholesome, delicious foods that provide optimal fuel for physical activity and optimal flavor for satisfaction. You'll be amazed at how much you can eat with a Mile-High Metabolism and still stay lean.

We've seen other diet experts urge people to become vigilant about their diet and physical activity program, but Coloradans (and people in the NWCR) have taught us that this is a backward approach. Yes, people who succeed at weight loss and healthy living *do* spend a lot of time thinking about healthy eating and physical activity. Yet it's not from a place of anxiety or a desire to be "good." Rather, they relish and look forward to these things. The key to success is savoring this lifestyle and doing it in a way that brings you happiness rather than a feeling of hardship. We know this is possible, because we've seen it in our friends, neighbors, and colleagues and in people across the country who have succeeded in losing weight and keeping it off.

Sure, you'll have to restrict your calories temporarily to drop pounds, but if you adopt the Colorado lifestyle, this will be a short-term fix, not a forever reality. Get the weight off and adjust your metabolism, and you can live in a healthy, enjoyable way and stay satisfied and slim. You can even have indulgence meals where anything you want is on the table. However, your idea of what's indulgent might change. We've found that over time, people lose the desire for things they once thought they could never live without. Yes, they actually learn to like and prefer healthier foods.

By the time you've completed the Colorado Diet, we're confident that you will feel this way, too. The steps outlined in the chapters that follow will help you reach your weight goal gradually, without ever feeling deprived. By the end, you may be surprised to find that our Colorado plan no longer feels like a diet but is simply your new favorite way of living.

———

Ours isn't the first plan to promise permanent weight loss. But how many plans can back up those claims with results from research involving thousands of real people? Our claims are based on the achievements of participants in the NWCR across the country, the patients in our weight-loss clinic, and the residents of Colorado who are lean and living the lifestyle we will help you adopt. The Colorado Diet works—we see the evidence of its success every day.

The Mile-High Metabolism

CHAPTER 2

EVER NOTICE HOW SOME people can pile an extra slice of lasagna on their plate or help themselves to a heaping piece of cake and never have trouble zipping up their jeans? Those surplus calories they eat here and there *should* add up to several pounds of weight gain over the course of a year, and yet these lucky souls maintain a near-constant number on the scale. They don't skip their next meal or pull out a calculator to tabulate how many miles they need to walk to burn off the chocolate cheesecake. So how do they do it? They've maintained a Mile-High Metabolism.

The word *metabolism* gets tossed around a lot, but most people aren't sure what it means. Put simply, metabolism is the process by which the body converts food to energy it can use. It's the sum of all the chemical reactions and physical processes that occur in our bodies—from hormone production, to digestion, to pumping blood, to breathing, to walking, and more. Even when you're asleep or

13

sitting completely still, your body needs energy to keep it going, so your metabolism is active around the clock.

In an ideal world, your metabolism adapts to your diet. You burn all the calories you consume, regardless of whether they come from protein, carbohydrate, or fat, and if you eat a little more or less on any given day, your metabolism compensates by speeding up or slowing down. That's what we call a Mile-High Metabolism—one that quickly adjusts to your calorie intake and activity level. The human body is built to move, and it needs high-octane fuel to function at its best. When your body stops moving as it was intended to or if you supply it with inferior fuel, your metabolism begins to deteriorate. You become more efficient at *storing* calories, in the form of body fat, than burning them.

The Colorado Diet repairs your metabolism so that you can stop stockpiling fat and prevent those unwanted pounds from creeping up on you.

YOUR BODY, THE BATHTUB

Imagine for a moment a bathtub with a clogged drain and the faucet turned on full blast. Your body is the tub. Water (or the calories you eat) gushes into the tub faster than it can clear the drain (your metabolism, or the calories you burn). As a result, the water level in the tub (your weight) increases.

Most diet plans focus on reducing the amount of water that flows into the tub by slowing the faucet to a trickle (restricting food intake). That works for a while. Eventually, though, the water level begins to creep up again—slowly if you keep the faucet on low, but very quickly if you happen to turn the knob higher. Why? Because the drain is clogged. However, if you fix the drain while the faucet is on low, you can reduce the tub's water level and later turn the faucet back up and still keep the water level low.

To get to a healthy weight and stay there, you have to completely revamp your tub. That requires three things:

1. Turning the faucet down *temporarily* so the water level is lowered

2. Unclogging your drain and increasing its diameter so water flows more freely—even when the tap is on full blast

3. Adjusting your faucet to match your drain's capacity and keep it clear

Using this bathtub analogy, having a Mile-High Metabolism means your drain (metabolism) automatically responds to the amount of water (food) coming in so the water level in your tub (your weight) stays steady.

The ability to adjust to your changing food intake and switch between carbohydrates and fat for energy is known in scientific circles as "metabolic flexibility." Genetics plays a role in metabolic flexibility, just as it does in height and eye color. Some people, such as the "easy gainers" we describe in "What's Your Metabolism Personality?" (page 26), are naturally more likely to drift into fat-storage mode than others, while those skinny kids who can't for the life of them gain weight are genetically programmed to maintain a high level of metabolic flexibility. But the good news is that unlike height and eye color, metabolic flexibility is a trait that you can influence with your behavior. Everyone has the capacity to develop a Mile-High Metabolism.

GETTING OUT OF FAT-STORING MODE

The overall result of an inflexible metabolism is that your body hoards most of the fat you eat in your fat cells. (So when people say ice cream goes straight to their hips, they aren't exaggerating!) This is what we mean when we say your body is stuck in fat-storing mode.

You often hear that extra protein and carbohydrate calories are converted to fat. Except under extremely rare circumstances, this isn't true. So what happens to the carbohydrate and protein you eat? No matter how much of these two nutrients you consume, you can only store a tiny amount of each. All of the rest is burned. That does not mean that you can eat as much of them as you want, though. If you have a surplus of carbohydrate and protein, your body will use them at the expense of fat. They may not turn into fat, but they *shut off fat-burning.*

To understand how, you need to know how the body uses two hormones, insulin and leptin. Carbohydrate, and to a lesser extent protein, stimulates the pancreas to produce insulin. Insulin's job is to shuttle glucose (the end product of carbohydrate digestion) from the bloodstream into cells where it can be used for energy or stored as muscle glycogen (the liver can also store some glycogen). It also promotes uptake of amino acids from protein digestion into muscle cells to support normal muscle repair. (Any excess amino acids are burned for fuel.) Your body will not burn fat while your insulin level is high. It's focused on using glucose. But once all of the glucose and glycogen is used, the insulin level falls and fat is readily released from your fat cells to keep your body going until your next infusion of glucose.

When you overconsume protein and carbohydrate, though, your insulin level never gets low enough and your body doesn't get a chance to tap into its fat stores. What's more, any fat you do eat is shuttled directly into your fat cells for storage, adding to the fat that's already there—and you gain weight.

(You can't get around this by cutting all fat out of your diet. First, for practical purposes it's impossible. The vast majority of foods are some combination of protein, carbohydrate, and fat. For instance, while beef is mostly protein, even lean cuts have *some* fat. Avocados and nuts are mostly fat, but they also contain protein and carbohydrate. But even if you were able to reduce your fat intake to zero, your body would convert excess carbs to fat, that being one of the extremely rare circumstances we mentioned above.)

If you have a Mile-High Metabolism, you never get to this point, thanks to the action of leptin. Fat cells produce this hormone when fat storage is adequate to signal the brain to reduce appetite. You feel full, you stop eating, your insulin levels drop, and your body burns some of its stored fat. Fat cells then need to be replenished, so they stop making leptin and that stimulates appetite.

If you override leptin's signal and keep eating, your fat cells get larger and produce even more leptin in an effort to get your brain to stop you. Keep ignoring leptin's call, though, and the communication loop breaks down. Your brain becomes resistant to leptin—the signal to reduce food intake is there but the brain doesn't recognize it—and appetite increases. Your body is no longer in harmony, and your metabolism has become inflexible.

EXERCISE IS YOUR DRANO

Understanding metabolic flexibility should help you recognize why just turning down the spigot (eating less) alone does not lead to long-term weight loss. You can lose weight this way, but simply losing weight does not fix your inflexible metabolism. As your body decreases in size, the number of calories it takes to maintain your weight also decreases. It's simple physics: It takes more energy to move a larger mass than it does to move a smaller one. The bigger your body size, the more energy you need just to maintain your body functions. A 200-pound person will burn about 225 more calories at rest each day than a 150-pound person. And that same 200-pound person will burn about 100 more calories in an hour of walking than a 150-pound person because it takes more energy to move a heavier object.

The kind of food restriction required to maintain a lower body weight is unsustainable—and you can't keep turning down the spigot forever. Your body is programmed to operate with an open spigot. Humans have a strong biological instinct to eat a lot of food because a few thousand years ago, food was more scarce and our ancestors had to work hard to obtain it. As a result, we developed a tendency to eat our fill when food is available and to store extra energy by building up our fat reserves so we'd have resources when there wasn't much around to consume. Our lifestyles and eating habits have changed enormously since then, but the human body has not. Restricting food, especially when there's plenty of it available, is something that we simply aren't programmed to do.

When you stop moving, buildup begins in your drain: Metabolic harmony is gradually disrupted, and your metabolism becomes less and less flexible. Eventually, your drain clogs. Muscles become resistant to insulin, so their ability to switch from carbohydrate to fat as a fuel source slows. The number of mitochondria—the power centers of cells that convert carbohydrate and fat to energy—in muscle tissue declines. There is also a reduction in those muscle fibers that burn fat best. The body tries to compensate for muscle insulin resistance by pumping out more insulin. This inhibits fat release and triggers fat storage. The result is larger fat cells.

In our weight loss clinic, we tell people that if they aren't prepared to increase their movement substantially, their chances of being successful over the long term are low. Losing weight without increasing physical activity makes it practically impossible to relax your diet vigilance even a little. When you are physically active, you burn the fuel you take in. The spigot is wide open, but so is your drain, so very little water builds up in the tub. And that's how people pretty much lived until the mid-20th century, when our drains started to get "clogged" as we slowed our physical activity.

Even the decline in activity levels over just a few generations has made a difference in our metabolisms. A study led by Dr. Tim Church at the Pennington Biomedical Research Center looked at changes in physical activity in the workplace from the 1960s to the present. He calculated that today's sedentary workers expend 140 to 160 fewer calories per day in physical activity than office workers of the past. Overall, the amount of physical activity required for the routine tasks of daily living (such as washing dishes and clothes, preparing meals, mowing the grass, and getting from point A to point B) is less than it used to be, in great part due to technology. But there's one group of Americans who still live the way we did at the start of the 20th century: the Amish.

People in Amish communities lead lifestyles that resemble a typical American's lifestyle in the late 19th and early 20th centuries. They walk most places or drive horse and buggies and farm in a way that relies on human power. The Amish eat a diet very much like the one most people ate 100 years ago—meat, potatoes, homegrown vegetables, and homemade pies and other baked goods. It's obviously not a low-calorie diet, yet obesity rates in these communities are extraordinarily low: *zero* for men and just 4 percent for women.

What's the Amish secret? It's their active lifestyles. Dr. David Basset Jr. at the University of Tennessee found that in a typical day, the Amish men walk an average of 18,000 steps (about 8 miles), while Amish women get 14,000 steps (more than 6 miles). All that activity gives them the metabolic flexibility to burn what they eat and helps regulate appetite so their bodies tell them when to stop eating naturally. This is the way everyone's body was intended to work, but most people don't move enough to keep their metabolism running properly.

It doesn't take very long for a lack of movement to begin to clog your drain. Dr. Audrey Bergouignan, our colleague at the University of Colorado, showed just how quickly it happens. She reviewed 60 years of research on bed rest—and that's about as sedentary as you can get! In these studies, active people volunteered to undergo complete bed rest for periods that ranged from a few days to several months. What Dr. Bergouignan learned was amazing. People's metabolisms began losing flexibility after just a *single day*. Now imagine what 10 years of inactivity can do to your metabolism.

GET YOUR APPETITE IN THE REGULATED ZONE

Exercise keeps your metabolism flexible, but it also it keeps your appetite balanced. Psychologist John Blundell at the University of Leeds has labeled the metabolic circumstance where you're active enough to balance your food intake and energy needs as the "regulated zone." When you're in the regulated zone, your body is working with you to achieve a healthy weight. Without exercise, your appetite becomes uncoupled from your body's energy needs. The result? You can eat more than your energy needs.

Studies in the 1950s by Tufts University scientist Jean Mayer were the first to reveal this paradox. Dr. Mayer examined food intake and body weight across a range of occupations, in hundreds of people from sedentary office workers to farmers and laborers. Without any deliberate calorie counting, workers in jobs that required some physical activity matched their food intake to their energy demands, so their weight stayed healthy and stable.

But here's where it gets interesting. Mayer found that people in the most sedentary occupations ate far more calories than they needed to meet the energy demands of their jobs, and these workers were much more likely to be overweight and obese. The message was clear. People whose daily lives required physical activity maintained precise appetite control and food intakes, while those living a sedentary lifestyle did not adjust their food intake downward to match their tiny energy expenditures—and they gained weight.

SURPRISE: YOU DO NOT NEED TO EXERCISE TO *LOSE* WEIGHT

Given that we just spent several pages explaining why exercise is so crucial to fixing your metabolism, this statement may shock you: Adding physical activity to a food-restricted diet does not really produce that much more weight loss. Our colleague Dr. Rena Wing at Brown University found this when she reviewed studies involving weight loss with diet (food restriction) alone versus diet and exercise. There was very little difference in weight loss between the two approaches. How can this be? Weight loss is determined by the "negative energy deficit," which is the difference between how many calories you take in and how many you burn. Most people find it easier to eat 500 calories fewer than to move 500 calories more. Think of it— you can cut 500 calories simply by having a smaller meal, but a 170-pound person would need to walk for about 90 minutes to burn the same 500 calories. It's not that exercise can't produce weight loss, it's just that it requires much more time and effort than eating less.

A PARADOX

Modern life is notoriously sedentary, so you'd expect that desk jockeys would have much lower daily energy (calorie) expenditures than our nomadic ancestors or populations who still require lots of exercise for daily living. But it turns out that this isn't the case. Recent research shows that the number of calories that today's hunter-gatherer people burn each day is about equal to the calories sedentary office workers burn. Yet those populations are lean and fit and our contemporary American population is fat and unhealthy.

How can this be? It turns out that active and sedentary people reach a similar level of energy expenditure by two very different paths—being physically active or by gaining weight. Here's how it works: We previously explained that if you gain weight, you require more calories just to keep your now bigger body alive. Your body wants to consume a lot of food, and there are really only two things it can do with these calories—burn them or store them. If you move more, you burn more; if you're sedentary, the extra calories result in weight and fat gain. As your weight increases, you burn more calories. This is because it takes more energy to maintain and move a bigger body than a smaller one. This is the way our modern bodies have developed to burn the calories we are eating without doing more exercise. Modern hunter-gatherers move more and store less, and consequently, they're lean, smaller people. Typical sedentary Americans, on the other hand, store more calories and gain weight to get to the same level of total energy expenditure as our active hunter-gatherer ancestors without doing all the movement.

However, you *must* exercise to keep the weight off. Lasting weight loss is really a two-part process. Step one is to temporarily turn down your spigot (eating less) to bring the water level (your body weight) down. But if the drain is still clogged, the water level will inevitably rise again.

Step 2 is to clear your drain—boost physical activity—so it can handle a stronger flow of water. According to our research and our analysis of data in the National Weight Control Registry, physical activity level is the best predictor of who will be successful in keeping weight off. Movement will fix your metabolism. This doesn't happen with just a few exercises sessions—typically it takes about 16 weeks—but the more active you are, the better your metabolism will function.

By developing a Mile-High Metabolism, you avoid having to restrict your food intake permanently. Once your drain is open, you can turn up the spigot. You can maintain your weight loss with a diet that is reasonable and filling. Yes, you have to learn to eat smarter, but you don't have to spend all day being hungry and counting calories.

A TALE OF TWO DIETERS

To illustrate the concepts we've been discussing, let's consider two hypothetical people who want to lose weight, Jessica and Rebecca. Both women are 45 years old and at their heaviest weight ever—225 pounds. Their weight and their lack of energy make it difficult for them to keep up with their kids. Their blood pressure and blood glucose levels are elevated to the point where their doctors say they'll need medication if they don't lose weight. After trying numerous diets over the years, they each decide that this year will be different and they pledge to lose weight by eating better and exercising for the rest of their lives. They are willing to do whatever it takes. On January 2, they start two very different weight-loss plans. See if you can spot the critical differences between the two strategies. More important, whose path would you like to follow?

Jessica's Path

Jessica chooses a diet plan that promises quick, easy weight loss. She takes in 1,000 fewer calories per day than she had been eating and loses about 2 pounds a week. Because her body is getting smaller, the number of calories she burns in her typical day also decreases. Her diet book mentions she should try to exercise some every day, but she really doesn't have time for that. Besides, she is losing weight at a good rate without it. In 8 weeks, she's down to 209 pounds. She's a little hungry, but she has more energy, and she's so happy with her weight loss that she vows to stick with her diet plan until she loses at least 35 more pounds.

Around this time, though, her weight loss slows. She discovers that she has to eat even fewer calories than she currently eats to lose any additional weight, and it's not easy. She spends a lot of time every day thinking and worrying about what she eats.

The next 5 pounds take several weeks to come off, and the next 2 pounds take even longer. After about 4 months, her weight is officially "stuck" at 202 pounds. She's hungry all the time. Her willpower fades, and she starts to eat "off" her diet plan—just a few bites here and there.

(continued on page 30)

WHAT'S YOUR METABOLISM PERSONALITY?

Hundreds of patients have come through our weight-loss clinic, and we've noticed that their weight troubles almost always trace back to the fact that their diets and their metabolism are not in sync. Here are three types of people we see frequently. Chances are, you'll see yourself in one of these real-life stories of "broken metabolism."

The Easy Gainer:
I have to eat perfectly to lose weight and keep it off

Joanne walked into our office carrying months of meticulous food diaries logging every bite she'd ever put in her mouth. Over the previous 3 months, she'd lost 30 pounds, but instead of feeling ecstatic, she was worried. She'd been here before. She would religiously follow a diet and the pounds would peel off, but the moment she allowed herself even a small indulgence—the second she so much as set eyes on a cookie—she'd gain it right back. She'd returned from a recent vacation 10 pounds heavier than when she'd left. She wanted to slim down, but she was tired of having to track every morsel. It seemed that she never had time to think about anything but food.

We call dieters like Joanne the "easy gainers." Their metabolism lacks any flexibility at all, so their bodies pack every single extra calorie onto their hips (or butts or bellies). For them, losing weight requires extra effort—more so than some of their peers. (It's unfair, we know.) Easy gainers have super-inflexible metabolisms. It's much harder for their bodies to turn on fat-burning simply by cutting back on what they eat. Joanne's 10-pound weight gain over a 2-week vacation is typical for people like her, most of whom have struggled with weight problems since childhood.

Joanne was on the verge of giving up when she came to us. She was tired of being hypervigilant about the food she ate and knew that something was wrong with her metabolism—and she was right! But her situation was far from hopeless. What she needed was a metabolism transformation. By moving her body and by learning to eat smarter, she was able to maintain her weight loss without having to spend every waking hour thinking about food.

The Healthy Over-Fueler:
I eat so healthy but never lose weight

Paula is a high school teacher, happily married with two young, active children. Her husband and kids are slim and healthy, but Paula struggled to lose the 20 pounds she'd gained with the birth of her last child. It wasn't for lack of trying. Making healthy meals for her family was a top priority, and Paula is well versed in nutrition. When we asked her to recall the foods she'd prepared over the previous weeks, she recited a long list of healthy items—whole grain breads, brown rice, fish, grilled chicken, almonds, natural peanut butter, berries, hummus, olive oil, walnuts, and lots of vegetables. She banned sugary soft drinks and favored whole foods over processed ones. Her occasional treats consisted of low-fat frozen yogurt or pudding. Paula wasn't supersizing her portions, and her family limited meals out to

(continued)

once per week. The whole family enjoyed physical activity together on the weekends, and Paula walked several times a week with some ladies in her neighborhood. She felt her lifestyle was pretty good, but her weight would not budge.

We see lots of people like Paula—we call them the "healthy over-fuelers." They're frustrated, and rightfully so. They're doing almost everything right—they're eating the right kinds of foods and engaging in some exercise. The level of water in their tubs is not going up, but it's not going down either. Their weight is stable but higher than they like.

Paula's problem was that she had mastered the art of weight maintenance, but she'd skipped the weight-loss step. Her moderate level of physical activity kept her metabolism from being too inflexible. But she was stuck, and to get unstuck we recommended phases 1 and 2 of the Colorado Diet. Paula needed to limit the amount of water flowing into her tub and to open the drain a little more by increasing her physical activity. She lost weight on the Colorado Diet, and then she went back to her healthy eating (which she had already turned into a habit). Increasing her physical activity to 70 minutes a day made it possible for her to maintain the lower body weight she achieved.

The Aging Gainer:
I can no longer eat whatever I want and stay lean

Tom walked into our office a few days after his 50th birthday. With an exasperated look on his face, he lifted his shirt and pinched a layer of fat on his belly. Up until a few years ago, he said, there was a six-pack where that roll of fat now hung over his waistband. In his twenties and thirties, Tom could eat whatever he wanted and never worry about his weight. He was moderately physically active but never felt that he had to go out of his way to make sure he hit the gym every day. Tom had never thought much about his lifestyle. Maintaining a healthy weight was something that happened without much effort. Then he turned 45, and it was like a switch flipped. Suddenly, his body stockpiled every extra calorie and stuffed it into the bulges of fat that kept covering up muscles that used to be visible.

Tom represents what we call the "aging gainers." It's an unfortunate fact of life that as you get older, your muscle mass naturally begins to decrease—by 5 to 10 percent per decade after about age 40. Consequently, the number of calories you burn decreases, and many people tend to put on some fat. While exercise can help reduce loss of muscle with aging, exercise can't prevent it totally. It's a process that happens so gradually that you may not notice it until one day, like Tom, you wake up with a pot belly.

A sluggish metabolism may feel like an added insult to an aging body, but unlike thinning hair, it's a problem you can do something about. The solution involves changes to both physical activity and diet. Even though Tom considered himself active, he had to ramp it up a little more. His natural Mile-High Metabolism was naturally slowing down. Adding more exercise helped limit the decline, but now he had to pay attention to his diet. His aging metabolism no longer allowed him to eat anything he wanted. He had to learn to eat smarter to match his diet to his changing metabolism. With this strategy, Tom lost 15 pounds, shed his spare tire, and regained his flat belly. He had to pay more attention to his lifestyle than before, but it was worth it.

Over the next 6 months, Jessica tries to eat well, but slowly she regains some of the weight she lost. That frustrates her because she really doesn't believe she is eating very much. She thinks she should be able to eat a slice of pizza every now and then, but it seems as though anything she puts in her mouth that is not "perfect" causes her to gain weight. Sometimes, she throws in the towel and eats whatever she wants. She begins to think she was just not meant to be lean.

Rebecca's Path

Rebecca chooses the Colorado Diet and jumps in. The book shows her how to eat smarter, and in phase 1 of the plan, she cuts 1,000 calories from her typical diet just by eating the foods in the portions listed. Because Rebecca's body (like Jessica's) is getting smaller, the number of calories she burns in her typical day also decreases. But at the same time, she starts to gradually increase her physical activity level both by walking for exercise and by moving around more during her everyday life. She moves on to phase 2 of the plan, where she has more food choices, and she ramps up her activity level slowly as outlined each week. At first, finding time for activity is hard, but she sticks with the plan, and it becomes easier over time to build it into her busy day. She's pleased that she's not hungry, the way she had been on previous diets. She drops 25 pounds over 8 weeks. She now weighs 200 pounds. She feels great but would like to lose more. She vows to stick to her plan and moves into phase 3 of the Colorado Diet.

On phase 3, her food choices become more varied again, and she gets to have some treats. This keeps her confidence and her determination high. She loses another 15 pounds in the next 8 weeks. After about 4 months, she weighs 185 pounds. She is surprised to see that she is eating about the same number of calories as she was eating before her weight loss, but now she is eating much better food. She now also gets about 70 minutes of activity a day, and she's burning a significant number of calories.

Rebecca continues to eat smarter and exercise over the next 6 months. She is energized and has created a new life for herself. She joined a gym and really likes the Zumba classes. She starts a walking group with three other women in her neighborhood. She begins each day by thinking about how she will meet her exercise goal that day. She feels satisfied because she can eat a lot of good food and can have an occasional treat. When she notices her weight creeping back, she returns to phase 1 for a few days. She finally feels that she has the right tools to manage her weight forever.

––––––

So what happened here? Since Jessica did not ramp up her activity, she did not fix her broken, inflexible metabolism. Consequently, she tends to store fat easily when she overeats even a little bit, and when she tries to be good, she's hungry. She succeeded in losing weight, but she put herself in a situation where she had to maintain her weight loss on too few calories. Just to stay at 202 pounds, she will have to manage hunger forever, a scenario most people find unsustainable. Most people can't eat this way for more than about 6 months, and then their inflexible metabolism overpowers their determination and—guess what—the weight they worked so hard to lose is regained.

Rebecca, on the other hand, feels satisfied because she can eat a lot of good food and can have an occasional treat. Not only did she lose weight, she changed her lifestyle so the weight stays off. She has achieved a Mile-High Metabolism, which means she has metabolic flexibility and enhanced capacity to burn rather than store fat. As long as she eats smart and continues to meet her activity goal of 70 minutes of activity per day, 6 days a week, she will not regain her lost weight.

The Colorado Diet allows you to lose weight and end up with a Mile-High Metabolism and a lifestyle you can sustain forever. Now it's your choice: Do you want to be a Jessica or a Rebecca?

Prepare for Success:
The Colorado Mind-Set

MANY PEOPLE ENTHUSIASTICALLY JUMP into a weight-loss plan and promise themselves *this* time will be different. But just as many begin with trepidation, *hoping* that this time will be different, but not counting on it. Would it surprise you to hear that both "types" have equally strong odds of failure? In their excitement, the gung-ho people often neglect to plan adequately for the changes they need to make in order to succeed. And those who fear that they'll be hungry, that exercise will be too hard, or that they're destined to be heavy are adopting a self-fulfilling prophecy.

Our experience studying the lean people of Colorado and successful weight-loss maintainers around the country has shown us that an optimistic attitude balanced with a realistic understanding of how to make specific lifestyle changes—what we call a Colorado Mind-Set—is the most powerful tool for success. That's why before you alter your diet in any way or lace up your walking shoes, we want to help you develop and *sustain* the Colorado state of mind.

Notice the emphasis on *sustain*. Remember how in Chapter 2 we said that long-term weight loss is a two-step process? Taking the time to create a healthy mind-set at the start of your plan is a smart investment in your future. Not only does having a positive perspective make it easier for you to take the necessary first steps to lose weight, but the right attitude is essential for weight maintenance. Through our research, we've identified four strategies that help you develop a Colorado Mind-Set.

1. Find your motivation
2. Expect success
3. Make healthy decisions automatic
4. Create a supportive environment

1 / Find Your Motivation

Take a moment to reflect on your reasons for losing weight. Is it to fit into a smaller dress or to look good at your class reunion? To avoid developing diabetes or heart disease? To be able to walk up a flight of stairs without huffing and puffing? Maybe it's all these factors and more. These reasons are your "whys"—your impetus for sticking with your healthy lifestyle when things get tough—so you need to identify them clearly. Before you read any further, write them down—now. Your list can be as long or as short as you'd like, and there are no wrong whys. But you don't want to skip this step.

Now consider your purpose in life. We know—this sounds a bit heavy for a weight-loss book, but self-evaluation is crucial because understanding how losing weight relates to your purpose can generate some powerful whys. Ask yourself: "What is most important to me? What do I hope to accomplish in the next 5, 10, 15 years and beyond?" Perhaps you want to be the best parent, grandparent, or role model possible. You might aspire to become a serious musician or the CEO of your company. Or you might desire to help children learn to read, advocate for animals, be a famous author or actor, or serve our country in the military—or a combination of these. There is no wrong or right purpose—all that matters is that you identify yours. Write your purpose at the top of your list of whys for weight loss. (If you're having trouble identifying your purpose, don't worry—you can still start the Colorado Diet. Often, your purpose emerges as you begin to lose weight. We'll give you exercises to identify and refine your purpose in every phase of the Colorado Diet.)

Next, consider how living a healthy lifestyle and losing weight will assist you in achieving your purpose. For instance, will being leaner and healthier increase your chance of avoiding the heart disease that runs in your family? If so, how might that tie back to your purpose? Will it help you attain your goal of seeing your grandchildren grow up? Will having more energy make it easier for you to do the work necessary to climb to the top of the corporate ladder? Maybe your purpose is to educate children by writing children's books, and living a healthier lifestyle gives you the confidence to pitch your ideas to a publisher. Perhaps making lifestyle changes for your health allows you to nurture yourself and pay attention to your own needs after years of looking after others. Now ask yourself: Are your current weight and lifestyle helping or standing in the way of realizing these objectives?

In thinking about how your new lifestyle and weight loss will

HOLLY'S PURPOSE

My purpose in life has always been to help people lose weight. It's what I think about in the middle of the night, it's what I study, it's what I do in my clinic, it's what I write about. I'm sure it's what I was meant to do, and I'm blessed that my life and career took me down a path that allows me to achieve my purpose. As I mentioned in Chapter 2, I'm an "easy gainer." I gain weight at the drop of a hat if my activity level falls. I follow the Colorado Diet, too. It's the only plan I know of that keeps my metabolism in good working order and allows me to maintain a healthy weight. But I sometimes struggle to stick with my plan. When I do, I recall my purpose, and that motivates me to continue my healthy lifestyle. I have a strong internal need to be authentic and live my life with integrity. When I live by the Colorado Diet plan and maintain a healthy weight, I feel authentic, honest, and genuine. I'm practicing what I preach—not just telling my patients what *they* should do—and it makes *me* feel good. That doesn't mean I never have an ice-cream cone or skip a workout. But if I stray from the Colorado Diet for long, life doesn't feel right. I feel like a hypocrite, and that often leads to other negative emotions. I don't connect with my patients as well, and that means I'm not doing my job properly. Your internal motivator, your purpose, may be different, but once you find it, it will be no less powerful. Spend some time thinking about what keeps you going. Trust me, you won't regret it.

help you achieve your purpose, you might discover a few powerful whys that hadn't occurred to you earlier. Add these to your list and star them. Also put a star next to any other reasons for losing weight that are related to your purpose. Maybe they all are. These are your deeper whys. Because they're related to your purpose, they're more likely to be a continued source of motivation, even after you have lost the excess weight. They're what will motivate you after people have stopped complimenting you on your success and after you fit into your favorite pair of jeans. Your goal is to use your new healthy lifestyle as a means to an end. And the end needs to be something that's important to *you*, not to your neighbor, your spouse, or your best friend.

Not all your whys have to relate directly to your purpose, though. Maybe your top why right now is to win a weight-loss contest at work, not to have to pay extra money for health insurance because you are overweight, or to fit into a special outfit for a class reunion or a wedding. These external whys are perfectly legitimate. They provide motivation in the short term. For lasting success, though, strive to connect your whys and your purpose, because internal whys (those related to your purpose) are more powerful incentives. For instance, studies by Dr. Pedro Teixeira, a behavioral psychologist from Portugal, have found that people with internal motivation do much better at staying with an exercise program than those with external motivation. But he also discovered that those who started with external motivators and *switched* to internal ones did just as well as those who began with the internal types.

Our research shows that whys evolve over time. As you lose weight, some whys will probably disappear and new ones will develop.

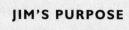 **JIM'S PURPOSE**

Earlier in my life, my purpose was to become the best scientist I could be and discover important things about human health. But what really excites me today is using what we learn from our research to help people achieve healthier, happier lifestyles. There's a lot of misinformation out there about how to lose weight and how to live a healthy lifestyle. Yet the situation isn't nearly as confusing as a lot of people believe. Experts know much more about the right ways to lose weight than we effectively communicate to the public. I truly believe that living an active, healthy lifestyle helps me do my job better. As with Holly, it's important for me to walk the talk. I can't claim that I'm too busy helping others to take care of myself. If I can't find the time to eat healthfully and exercise, how can I expect others to find time? Many of my whys relate to my purpose. I get so much pleasure from hiking and biking and skiing. I'm 62 years old, and, like my fellow baby boomers, I don't want to have to stop doing any of these things. I know that staying active and eating healthy gives me the best chance of continuing to live the life I love—and of achieving my purpose.

You may even discover that some whys that you initially thought were unrelated to your purpose actually are quite relevant. If you're struggling to link your reasons for weight loss to your purpose, think how you will feel once you achieve your weight loss. Many times, internal whys are related to feelings that result from achieving an external why. For example, you want to fit into size 10 jeans (external motivation) because . . . ? Because it will make you feel more confident (internal motivation). Has a lack of confidence kept you from going after the things you want in life? Perhaps the confidence you gain from fitting into a smaller size will transfer to other areas of your life and help you achieve your purpose.

Going forward, you'll refer to and adjust your list of whys frequently as you lose weight and continue to live the Colorado lifestyle. You'll add some motivators and delete others. Whenever you have a bad day and consider giving up your healthy lifestyle, recalling your deeper (internal) whys can keep you on your path. Your list provides the incentive to choose a smart breakfast most mornings instead of a quick doughnut or sugar-laden pastry. It spurs you to take a relaxing walk before dinner instead of plopping down on the couch in front of the TV. It reminds you to find extra time every day to move more without making excuses. It helps you stay the exercise course when it's cold outside or when your bike has a flat tire. It nudges you to eat smarter when you come home from a stressful day at work and pizza delivery is just a phone call away.

2 / Expect Success

Understanding your motivation is critical to your long-term success, but so is your mental approach to weight loss. Having the attitude that healthy living is a nourishing, happy, self-affirming way of life and thinking that eating healthy food and moving more are wonderful pleasures that you can look forward to every day—these are key elements of the Colorado Mind-Set. People with this frame of mind don't just strive to make healthy choices—eating healthy foods and engaging in physical activity are vital parts of who they are.

A "WHY" TRANSFORMATION

David came to us last year for help in losing weight. When we asked him why he wanted to slim down, he quickly replied: "I want to fit into a roller-coaster seat." He recalled the embarrassment and shame he felt on a recent trip to a theme park. His size had prevented him from taking his children on the roller coaster, and he believed that he had let his kids down. He quickly listed his goal as losing 70 pounds, and he indicated that fitting into a roller-coaster seat was one of his top motivations for doing it. We asked him to explain why sitting in a roller coaster was important and to imagine how he would feel when he did take the ride. He teared up. "I'll feel like a good father, one who can play with his kids and be a part of their lives and not hold them back. I'll feel strong and in control," he said. David has a powerful internal why lurking behind his external why. His extra weight was getting in the way of his purpose—being a good father. On the Colorado Diet, he dropped 60 pounds in 6 months. When the family took its next trip to the theme park, he rode the roller coaster with his children— and that was just the beginning of his journey. David became an assistant coach for his boys' soccer team, helping him further live a life connected to his purpose.

We find this same mind-set in people who have lost weight and kept it off (as well as in those who've never gained too much weight in the first place). And we find it in our successful patients, who, once they begin to eat healthfully and move their bodies, tell us that their whole approach to life has changed for the better.

Over the years, we've noticed that two types of patients come into our clinics: the defeatists and the optimists. Defeatists complain that adopting a new way of eating and exercising is just too hard. They harp that we're taking away all the fun and enjoyment in their lives. They often fixate on things they're missing out on and rant about how unfair it is. They have lists of excuses for why they can't follow the plan. They see us, not themselves, as responsible for their success. Defeatists might start a visit by saying, "I tried that step class you told me about, but the music was way too fast. I almost broke my ankle on one move. I quit halfway through the class, and I was sore for days. This isn't for me." Defeatists focus on the negative. They adopt a victim mentality.

Optimists come to our clinic focused on the benefits and opportunities presented by their new lifestyle. They usually start the visit recalling something wonderful they did that week or a barrier they overcame. They may tell us, "I tried that step class you suggested. It was a challenge, but I had fun. I laughed a lot, and even though the music was superfast, I made it through. Next time, I'll know what to expect, and I'll know to wear my other shoes. I was sore for a few days, but I guess that means I got a good workout and used muscles I haven't used in a while."

Optimists have a Colorado Mind-Set. They believe they have power over the things that happen to them, and they're inclined to put a positive spin on their experiences. They may struggle sometimes or feel sad about having to give up certain things, but they don't fixate on loss. Instead, they focus on finding solutions and ways to improve things.

In our clinic, the defeatist and the optimist follow the exact same diet and exercise program. Guess who loses more weight and gets the most out of their experience?

PRACTICE MAKES POSITIVE

Ronald came to our clinic desperate to lose weight. He was on oxygen and in a wheelchair most of the time because his knees and back could not support his 355 pounds. He arrived at the first appointment with his wife, and it was clear he was there at her insistence. Ronald told us all the reasons he had a weight problem— none of which were his fault. He lost his job and he hurt his knees, and so on. He used to have a really great life before all these terrible things happened to him and caused his weight to get out of control. Ronald was worried about his health, and that's why he wanted to lose weight. But he was not willing to change his current way of living to do so. He had a victim mentality. He finally agreed to start on a modified version of the Colorado Diet, but he absolutely refused to give up certain foods or to consider non-weight-bearing exercise in a pool. He referred to Holly as "Dr. Misery" and at every appointment would ask us what awful recommendations we had for him that day. Despite all that, he was able to drop about 30 pounds in

If your negative feelings about changing your lifestyle outweigh your positive ones, don't worry. Just as you worked to find your purpose, you can develop a sunnier attitude. Defeatists can become optimists. Many of our successful patients start out as skeptics, but at some point, they turn the corner, as we like to say. It's so gratifying to see this transition, because we know that it increases the chances of long-term success.

6 months, but we knew the weight would rebound if his mind-set didn't improve.

We wanted Ronald to drop the defeatist mentality, so we started each visit by asking him to name one good thing that had happened to him that week. We gave him "homework" designed to focus on the positives. It was slow going for him, and his visits became less frequent. Frankly, we weren't sure what would happen. Then one day, he came into our clinic after a 6-week absence, and he had lost another 20 pounds. He told us, "You know, some of those veggies you suggested I try taste pretty good if you grill them." We were speechless. He had finally visited the pool we had recommended months before. He went because he thought the warm water might feel good on his back. It took a while, but practicing to identify the positive benefits helped him turn the corner. These days, he can easily tell us things he is grateful for. He even stopped calling Holly "Dr. Misery." Today, he's down 90 pounds and is totally off oxygen. He sold his wheelchair on eBay.

How do you turn the corner and develop a Colorado Mind-Set? You practice focusing on the positives, not the negatives, of your new lifestyle by making conscious efforts every day to identify what you like about your new lifestyle and are grateful for. In each phase of the Colorado Diet, we give you exercises to guide you to a Colorado Mind-Set. You might have to work at this at first, but over time, your new, positive way of seeing the world will become natural.

3 / Make Healthy Decisions Automatic

In today's world, making healthy diet and physical activity choices takes planning and willpower. We're surrounded by unhealthy foods—and we have an innate preference for sugar, fat, and salt. Our lives are set up so we barely have to lift a finger to live them. Think of the number of fast-food restaurants in your neighborhood and the number of glowing screens (TVs, computers, smartphones) in your home. Choosing to live the Colorado lifestyle means sometimes passing on that dessert your taste buds are crying out for or finding a place to walk when you are on an out-of-town business trip and all you really want to do at the end of a long day of meetings is collapse in front of the TV. Sticking to your good intentions requires willpower in these circumstances.

Scientists who study willpower, such as Dr. Roy Baumeister, a psychologist at Florida State University, have found that the trait is like a muscle—it fatigues. And willpower doesn't come into play only when you're trying to make healthy choices: Controlling your temper, sticking to a budget, and working on that boring report all drain your reserves over the course of your day. As your willpower muscle tires, it becomes harder and harder to steer yourself away from a bad decision or resist temptation.

If you think of willpower as a finite resource, then you can learn to use it in the most efficient manner. The easiest way to stretch your willpower is to take it out of the equation: Plan ahead so that healthy choices become automatic and you don't have to rely solely on resolve. Studies show that people who make decisions ahead of time are far more likely to take action than those who leave things up in the air. For instance, you have a better chance of

<table>
<tr><td>

HOLLY'S TIPS

Start Early

</td><td>

When you bring home a bucket of fried chicken and plop down on the couch to veg out in front of the tube, it's often a sign that you've over-used your willpower muscle during the day. Many studies show that people have an easier time making healthy choices, like eating appropriate portions of food or going for a walk, first thing in the morning than they do in the evening. The same holds true for making better choices about eating and physical activity. So it's no surprise that so many people find that if they don't exercise first thing in the morning, they won't do it later in the day.

</td></tr>
</table>

picking a healthy, satisfying dinner at a restaurant if you peruse the menu online and decide what you'll order beforehand, rather than waiting to see what you feel like eating once you sit down at the table. This planning does not have to be extensive or time consuming. Preparing to eat healthfully may simply entail deciding which foods to keep out of the house, jotting down a shopping list of those foods, and then buying only the items on that list. Or you can treat exercise time like any other appointment—you just schedule it and go. You enter the time on your calendar and keep a gym bag with your workout clothes and gear at your office, in the trunk of your car, or wherever is most convenient.

When you do this over and over, the healthy behavior becomes a habit, a routine, or even a ritual. These terms are often

(continued on page 48)

PLANNING AND WILLPOWER

Jackie spent many years struggling with her weight—losing and gaining over and over. She weighed 175 pounds when she came to us. She never ate breakfast because she didn't feel hungry in the morning. Her first meal of the day would be a salad at lunch. By midafternoon, though, Jackie would be famished, and she'd dive into the snacks she kept in her desk—often fatty chips or sugary sweets. She knew that these weren't the healthiest options, but she told herself she needed them to get through her afternoon slump. As soon as she got home, she'd go directly to the refrigerator or cupboard for more snacks, and she'd nibble right up to dinnertime. She was so hungry and tired that she didn't have the energy to cook a healthy meal. The next thing she knew, she'd be sitting at the drive-thru window of a fast-food restaurant looking forward to some comfort food.

Jackie needed to better manage her willpower. Her eating patterns virtually ensured that she would need maximum willpower at the end of the day, when she was the most tired. Jackie started making progress when we convinced her that she should spread her calories over the day. She started eating breakfast but limited her choices to two healthy items. Those were the only breakfast foods she kept at home, so she never debated about whether to eat healthfully or not. Instead of using her willpower to skip breakfast, she was preserving it by designing a morning routine that was both healthy and easy. At work, she reduced her need for willpower by tossing the snack stash at her desk.

Since dinner was her biggest challenge, she reorganized her grocery shopping routine and started planning the evening meal in the morning, when her willpower was high. At the grocery store, Jackie bought whatever healthy protein source was on sale—fish, poultry, or meat, which was more economical in large packs. As soon as she got home from the market, she made it a habit to wrap the proteins into individual meal portions, which were easy to pop in the freezer. Then, each morning, the first thing she'd do was decide what to have for dinner, referring to a number of favorite core recipes she had developed for different types of fish, lean pork and beef, turkey, and chicken. She would write her dinner choice on her refrigerator note pad. Then she checked the fridge to see what veggies she had on hand and added those to her meal-planning list. Finally, she made sure she had the necessary herbs and spices. Before she left for work, she'd pull one of the individually wrapped packages of selected protein from the freezer so it would be thawed by the time she returned home. All she had to do in the evening was cook and assemble the meal she had already planned and committed to ahead of time. This saved a lot of decision making that would have been difficult in the evening, when her willpower was shot. She didn't always follow through on the healthy choice at dinner, but most of the time she found it easy to prepare what she'd planned.

Jackie stuck to this meal-planning routine. Over the next year, she successfully lost 35 pounds and kept it off. She found that planning a healthy dinner in the morning gave her something to look forward to. Rather than dreading the thought of having to make dinner, she was eager to get home to try out the new twists to her favorite recipes that she had come up with during the day.

used interchangeably. But while all of them help reinforce the new behaviors you're trying to establish, behavioral psychologists would say that habits, routines, and rituals are distinct.

Habits are patterns of behavior that are often subconscious—you do them without actively thinking about them—and triggered automatically by the environment in which you typically engage in that behavior. For instance, you've probably driven somewhere familiar in your car (for instance, to work) while having a fascinating conversation with the person in the passenger seat. Once you reach your destination, you realize you have no specific recollection of the journey itself, although somehow you navigated the exact route, obeyed traffic laws, and arrived safely. That's a habit—the brain has a "circuit" wired with the route from home to work that's cued by the landmarks along the way. You don't really have to "think" about how to get there. An example of a habit related to the Colorado Diet would be always choosing fat-free dairy products at the grocery store. Decide you are going to have only fat-free milk—no exceptions. Pretty soon, grabbing a gallon of fat-free milk will become automatic.

Routines are regular courses of action or procedure that accomplish some goal. They generally require more thought than habits do, but once you set them up, you don't need to think all that hard about them. For example, brushing your teeth may be part of your routine for getting ready for bed. Having something to eat before going to the grocery store so you aren't tempted by unhealthy foods is a routine.

Rituals are somewhat special: They are routines that typically have deeper meaning or symbolism beyond the immediate goal the behavior satisfies. Going to church on Sunday is a ritual because it fulfills a social and spiritual need. When it comes to weight loss, rituals are the routines you engage in that are connected to your deeper purpose. For example, dining at a healthy restaurant on Friday nights with friends is a ritual because along with a nice meal, you derive pleasure and connection from your relationships. Having a regular Saturday afternoon biking date with your child doesn't just get both of you moving, it serves to reinforce your purpose of being the best parent you can be.

As you follow the Colorado Diet, we want you to develop plans for your diet and physical activity and to create habits, routines, and rituals that lead you toward better choices so you can follow through on your intentions without tapping into your willpower. For example, you might plan to take your dog for a short walk every day first thing when you get home from work. Set a specific time for doing this and select the place you will go on your walk. Put the dog leash in a prominent place near the door to remind yourself that you have committed to do this. Put the walk on your calendar. The more often you take that walk, the more it will become automatic. It will become a routine or even a ritual (doing something for a good friend). The side benefit will be having the happiest dog in the neighborhood!

// *Building* Your Willpower

In the next few pages, we'll walk you through some common decision points you'll face as you go through the various phases of the Colorado Diet. Think about how you can plan ahead for these decisions and create new habits, routines, and rituals that will make the smart choices automatic. This process takes time, so go easy on

DEVELOPING A HEALTHY RITUAL

Trudy, a patient of Holly's, had a coffee date with her mom every Tuesday morning. They'd sit at a coffee shop for an hour, have a cup, and catch up. They both liked coffee, but the point was to spend time together regularly. One day, Trudy suggested that they meet at the mall so they could do a lap around the perimeter before sitting down to enjoy their coffee. The walk was a way for Trudy to create a ritual that reinforced her new healthy lifestyle and supported something that was important to her—spending time with her mom. It turns out that their time together felt more meaningful now, too, because they were doing something healthy for themselves—together.

yourself. The more you engage in a behavior, the less willpower you need and the easier the task becomes. It may take a few weeks or even months, but stick with the process, and positive change will happen.

Decision point: Grocery shopping

On each phase of the Colorado Diet, you're given a specific list of foods to choose from. But at the grocery store, you face unlimited choices. How do you ensure that you reach the checkout with the foods you're supposed to be eating now and not just the ones you're accustomed to buying? First, have a healthy snack before you shop so you can stave off impulses driven by hunger. Second, shop from your list and don't stray from it. Third, avoid the candy, soda, and snack food aisles. Now you have a healthy routine.

Decision point: Exercise

If you simply write "exercise" on your to-do list, you might never get to it. Instead, decide when to exercise, what type of activity you'll do, and where you'll do it. The more specific your plan, the better. Determine the time of day that exercise best fits into your schedule. This could be first thing in the morning—when your willpower muscle is strongest—during your lunch hour, or after work. It could be the same time every day or a different time, depending on the day. You might walk in the mornings on Mondays, Wednesdays, and Fridays; play tennis on Tuesday and Thursday evenings; and ride your bike on Saturday afternoons. Enter the activities on your calendar. Come up with ways to turn exercise time into a ritual by combining exercise with spiritual time or time with friends.

Decision point: Breakfast

Our research has shown that breakfast is an important meal. More than 95 percent of participants in the National Weight Control Registry are regular breakfast eaters. We want you to eat in the morning. Keep it simple by alternating among two to four different breakfasts—your morning meal choices can evolve as you move through the phases of the Colorado Diet. And don't just decide what to eat for breakfast; decide where you'll eat it—at home, at work, or in a restaurant. You can develop effective habits and routines to help keep breakfast healthy.

Consider the experience of our former patient Fred, who travels constantly in his job as CEO of a startup company. Before he came to our clinic, he would usually skip breakfast or just grab a doughnut and coffee. He insisted he didn't have time to research healthy breakfast options in all the places he travels. Fair enough. But there was a simple solution. He found that Starbucks serves oatmeal for breakfast—and there's a Starbucks everywhere. Now Fred heads to the nearest Starbucks every morning he is on the road and has oatmeal. It's easy. He doesn't have to expend any time, effort, or willpower about his a.m. meal.

Decision point: Lunch

The best way to ensure that you choose a healthy lunch is to prepare the meal at home ahead of time. Develop a set of three to five selections that you like and can easily make and turn these into your go-to lunches. You might plan a different lunch each day of the workweek—that's five different meals—and vary things on the weekend.

You can use the same strategy for lunches in a cafeteria or restaurant. Compile a list of go-to selections in advance, and then your only decision is which of these healthy choices you'll pick. Maybe you even plan out your lunch for every day of the week so that, for example, you hit the salad bar in the employee cafeteria every Wednesday.

Many of the people we work with have had success talking with the food service staff in their employers' cafeterias about providing healthier options. If you are looking for better food choices, chances are that many of your coworkers are as well.

Decision point: Snacking

A bag of chips staring you in the face is hard to resist. But if the only foods in your cupboards or fridge are the ones you decided to eat ahead of time, when your willpower was strong, it's almost impossible to make a bad choice. Stock your desk and your break room at work with healthy snacks, and your coworkers just might follow suit!

Decision point: Dining out

It's easier to stick to a healthy diet when you eat at home, because you have more control over what goes into your meals and your mouth. But restaurants are a part of life, and we want you to enjoy and feel comfortable eating at them. Dining-out decisions will depend on which phase of the Colorado Diet you are on. Frankly, it will be difficult to eat out during phase 1 (but remember—phase 1 lasts only 2 weeks). In phase 2, you can eat out, but you must select items that are included in your plan (more about this in Chapter 5). In phase 3, you have greater leeway to choose, but you still need to practice eating smarter.

With a little planning, you can dine out without undoing your progress. Study restaurant menus ahead of time (most places post theirs online) and look for items that fit with the plan. Often, you can consult an eatery's Web site to see how the dishes are prepared. Or ask the chef in person, before you place your order. In our experience, most are willing to discuss meal preparation with you.

TIPS FOR EATING SMARTER AT RESTAURANTS

- Avoid all-you-can-eat buffets.

- Watch portion sizes.

- Start your meal with a salad to help you avoid overeating.

- Drink water or unsweetened tea.

- Decline the bread or chips basket.

- Always ask for sauces and salad dressing on the side—use sparingly or bring your own.

- Select entrées that include vegetables.

- Remember, steamed, broiled, and grilled are better than fried.

- Tell your waiter that you do not use butter.

- Order an appetizer for a main course.

- Split an entrée with a friend or ask your server to put half in a take-away container.

- Order à la carte—such as a grilled lean protein (without butter or sauce) and veggies.

- Consider fruit for dessert.

- Don't be afraid to ask about ingredients or substitutions.

Decision point: Bedtime

Surprised to see this on the list? For many years, experts have been uncovering connections between sleep problems and weight gain, and a recent review of many of these studies published in the journal *Obesity* found a strong association. Sleep problems include sleep deprivation and not getting quality sleep (waking up frequently, having restless sleep, or feeling tired the next day). Researchers don't completely understand why people who experience inadequate sleep or who have poor sleep quality are more likely to be overweight than those who get 7 to 8 hours of solid shut-eye each night. Some studies suggest that sleep problems disrupt hormones

THE FRIENDSHIP FACTOR

Last year, Jim's son Alex moved from Colorado to Mississippi for work. In Colorado, his social life revolved around playing Ultimate Frisbee, hiking, and skiing with friends. In his new home, his social life revolved around food and drink. Alex gained about 20 pounds in the first 6 months. When he realized that his weight gain was the direct result of his new lifestyle, Alex decided to seek out friends who were more interested in healthy activities. He joined an Ultimate Frisbee team, began running, and started eating at home more often. He even encouraged his other friends and coworkers to move more. Alex has lost every extra pound and is back to his Colorado weight.

that are involved in appetite regulation (such as leptin and ghrelin), leading to increased appetite and greater food intake. There's also evidence that lack of sleep boosts cravings for foods high in sugar and fat. We believe another reason is that your willpower is weaker when you're tired, so you're more likely to give in to temptation and make poor diet and activity choices. On the other hand, scientists have shown that rest and sleep restore your willpower, in the same way rest helps an athlete's muscles restore to their peak performance. In Resources on page 227, we list some sites that will help you identify and address sleep issues.

4 / Create a Supportive Environment

You want your surroundings and your relationships to work for, not against, your efforts. People who lose weight and keep it off engineer their environments so that healthy choices for eating or physical activity are easily available and unhealthy ones are less accessible.

This could mean not having sugary soda, candy, cookies, or other similar foods in your house. If temptation isn't there, you can't give in to it. However, if you're truly hungry, you need to eat something, so keep plenty of tasty, healthy foods on hand so you don't miss the unhealthy ones. Store fresh fruit on your counter—it's a visual reminder to eat it. Keep veggie snacks like baby carrots, edamame, or bell pepper strips in zipper-lock bags so a quick grab-and-go munch selection is always within arm's reach. Convenience is the key here—if the food is ready to eat, it will fit the bill.

Go through your pantry, refrigerator, and freezer and eliminate as many of the sugary, starchy convenience foods that are high in fat and calories as you can—toaster pastries, ramen noodles, mac 'n' cheese, microwave burritos, frozen potpies, and the like. Swap these for the foods we recommend for each phase of the Colorado Diet. The purpose of this purge is not only to eliminate the unhealthy choices but also to have healthy foods right there, ready to go.

You can revamp your work environment as well. Are healthy snacks available? If not, bring your own to work. Maybe folks at your office routinely supply the gang with unhealthy snacks (we're all familiar with doughnut Fridays or office birthday parties with cake). Can you get them to change? If not, what routines can *you* change so that you don't have to partake? Perhaps rerouting your path to the photocopier or the restroom will divert you around the "temptation zone."

A parent who is trying to lose weight often thinks he or she needs to keep "special" foods (like cookies, chips, candy, etc.) in a special place for the rest of the family. This approach is a mistake. Creating a home food environment that limits the number of poor nutritional choices is a great strategy any family can use to ensure that everyone eats a healthy, balanced diet. Kids opt for convenience, just like adults, so having healthy grab-and-go snacks in resealable bags readily available—plus lots of fresh fruit peeled, cored, and cut up—will win you points with the young hungry hordes. It's no secret that kids in America today are experiencing more and more "adult" diseases like obesity and type 2 diabetes and showing the hallmark signs of premature heart disease risk. So, parents, think of this step as a way to create a healthy environment for your whole family.

Also consider ways you can tweak your environment to encourage you to be active. Many research studies have shown that the more time you spend sitting in front of a screen (TV, computer, video game), the more likely it is you'll gain weight. One Canadian study found that too much screen time increases the risk of obesity in children by 10 to 61 percent. Now, it would be silly to suggest getting rid of all screens. But just as you can overindulge on food, you can overindulge on screen time. Perhaps you can resolve not to have a TV in every room. Or you could set up a treadmill or stationary bike to use while watching television. You can even devise habits, routines, or rituals that help you avoid too much screen time. At our research center, we've posted a "step map" on the wall that lists all the local restaurants, coffee shops, and other attractions and how far they are, in steps, from our building. You could map your neighborhood hot spots, creating a chart showing the number of steps it takes to get to different shops, restaurants, etc. You can also develop a few specific walking routes so that when you want a 4,000-step walk after dinner, you know right where to go.

// *Building* Supportive Relationships

The people you interact with—at work, at home, and in your community—have a tremendous influence on your own behavior. In Colorado, for instance, you might feel left out if you *aren't* out hiking, biking, skiing, or walking. The social environment here promotes healthy living. People use physical pursuits like running and dancing as social events. If your friends are constantly organizing hikes and bike rides, you'll find it difficult not to go along at least some of the time. The more you can create a supportive social environment where you live, the easier it will be to maintain your desired lifestyle.

If you're not already surrounded by healthy, active people, don't worry. Our research shows that you can change your current environment even if healthy living isn't a big part of your current relationships. For example, Mark, one of the successful weight-loss maintainers we studied, initially gained weight because the people he socialized with went out to bars and restaurants most nights. Too much pizza and beer led him to gain 50 pounds. Adopting the Colorado Diet helped him drop those extra pounds, but he realized that if he wanted to keep the weight off, he couldn't go back to hanging out where food and drink was the focus. Mark went online to find a volleyball league in his neighborhood, and he now spends time with people who are active. He sees his old friends, too, but he avoids going to bars and restaurants with them. We encourage you to seek out people who are already active, and follow their lead. In Resources on page 227, we direct you to options for finding active social networks.

Of course, we don't want you to dump your family or friends, even if they're not engaged in a healthy lifestyle, but you do need to recognize the influence they have on your behavior. And consider this: Perhaps your improved behavior will rub off on them. Is there a friend or relative who might join you on your weight-loss journey? It can be uncomfortable to come out and say, "Hey, I need to lose weight, and you do, too. Want to do it together?" But you can ask friends or family members to join you on a walk or to grab a bite at a restaurant that serves healthful fare. Even if they don't choose to join you in your new lifestyle, they can support your choices.

REINFORCING CHANGE

Developing a Colorado Mind-Set takes some effort, but here's the good news. Once you begin the Colorado Diet, you will benefit from a positive feedback loop. Changes in your diet and exercise behaviors will directly lead to changes in your mood and even in the neural network of your brain. In turn, these brain changes make it easier to maintain improvements in diet and exercise. The physiological feedback loops will kick in automatically with the Colorado Diet, and many of the psychological ones will, too.

This is how that whole process works. By following the Colorado Diet, you shut off your cravings for sugary, high-calorie fare. Before long, your desire for those foods diminishes, and you're less tempted to indulge. Incorporating regular physical activity into your life doesn't just fix your metabolism, it also boosts your energy levels, helps you sleep better, and ups your overall sense of well-being. Physical activity has been shown to increase serotonin and other mood-improving chemicals in the brain. You may even start to crave the energized feeling and the spirit-lifting rewards that come from daily movement. Over time, your mind associates feeling good with exercise and a better diet, and that reinforces your healthy lifestyle.

When you engage in a new behavior, your brain creates new connections between brain neurons that didn't communicate with each other before. Keep using these new connections and they become "hardwired," so that a particular behavior becomes a habit. The more you continue to engage in healthy behaviors, the more they become hardwired, and your old, unused, unhealthy neural connections weaken. Add in the fact that you're losing weight and reaping the feel-good benefits that come from dropping those extra pounds, and you've got a powerful, self-reinforcing loop. The result? Your appetite is driven by your actual metabolic needs, not by unhealthy cravings. Your brain and your body work together in harmony. Your body burns fat. Your energy levels have never been higher. You feel great!

Prepare to Move:
The Right Way to Exercise

CHAPTER 4

BEING ACTIVE NEARLY EVERY day isn't optional. It's the key to developing a Mile-High Metabolism and the deciding factor that ensures the weight you lose on the Colorado Diet will be gone for good. That's why we want you eventually to be moving 70 minutes a day, six days a week.

If exercise hasn't been part of your routine, recently or ever, this may seem like an enormous challenge. You might be concerned about finding the time or worried that every minute you spend exercising will feel boring or difficult. Or maybe you think you've heard all this before—but we bet you haven't heard it presented exactly the same way we do in this chapter.

We take a detailed approach to helping you overcome your activity barriers, walking you through the process of building a plan step-by-step, and giving you a program to follow for each phase of the

Colorado Diet. We've found that when the steps are specific—and, just as important, when you contemplate what you'll need to do before jumping in—they get into your psyche in a way they haven't before and therefore have more lasting power.

A multitude of evidence backs up our observations. Studies show that "planning" for success when attempting to create change makes a big difference not just in increasing physical activity in people of all ages, but for a variety of healthy behaviors, from breast self-exams in women to flossing your teeth regularly. When it comes to exercise, the most compelling data on the value of planning come from research involving people who started out leading very sedentary lifestyles. One study implemented a "planning to be active" program that focused on getting people to write down what activities they were going to do as well as when and where they were going to do them. Compared with the control group that did not participate in the planning strategy, the members of the planning group increased the number of days they performed moderate to vigorous physical activity from less than 1 day per week to more than 3½ days a week. Another study published in the *American Journal of Preventive Medicine* reported that engaging in a consistent exercise plan doubled the chances of successfully maintaining an exercise program and keeping off weight.

BEFORE YOU START: USE SOME MENTAL MUSCLE

Most people who fail to stick to an exercise program do so because they weren't ready to start in the first place. They didn't consider it important enough to make it a priority, and they didn't have a plan for dealing with the barriers they would face. Just like planning makes a difference when you're setting up a business, hosting a party, or plotting out an amazing family vacation, a little exercise planning goes a long way toward ensuring a successful outcome.

To get yourself in an active mind-set, spend a few minutes writing down the pros and cons of adding movement to your life. For instance, consider that it will help you:

- Maintain your weight

- Live longer

- Keep your brain sharp as you age

- Eat more food without gaining weight

What about the cons? Here are ones we hear frequently:

- I don't have the time.

- Exercise hurts.

- I hate exercise.

- I don't know where to exercise.

- I'm not really convinced that I need to exercise to stay at a healthy weight.

Notice anything about the points on these lists—and probably on yours as well? Most of the pros focus on long-term payoffs, while most of the cons affect your life immediately. Although long-term benefits are important—and many of them help fulfill your purpose—it can take a while to see the fruits of your efforts. To make exercise a habit, concentrate on what being active can do for you *right now*. Regular exercisers report that they're motivated to exercise because it gives them more energy, improves their mood, reduces stress, boosts creativity, and allows them time for themselves or to be with family or friends. It may take a few sessions for you to notice these benefits, but as your muscles and your brain get used to moving, you, too, will see how pleasurable exercise can be.

Given busy schedules and environments that work against rather than for you, to incorporate physical activity successfully into your life you'll need some powerful pros and strong strategies for overcoming the cons. But we're confident that we can get you from where you are right now (even if it is sitting on the couch) to a place where you're moving 70 minutes a day, 6 days each week—and liking it. From our research, we see that people emphasize the pros and minimize the cons by asking themselves the following questions.

// Why do you want to become active?

You might expect that people with demanding jobs or many family obligations exercise less than those without these time constraints. Or you might believe that people with access to gyms or personal trainers or who live in communities with sidewalks have an easier time sticking to an exercise program. Yet that's not what our research has shown. What separates regular exercisers from sporadic ones is their commitment to making physical activity a priority. It's not enough to decide to give it a "try"—you'll probably fail with this attitude because you have not committed. Focusing on the pros of physical activity will give you that resolve. Think back to your purpose that you identified in Chapter 3. How will adding physical activity into your life help achieve it? Now recall the point we made in Chapter 2: Every part of your body—including your brain—works better when you are moving.

People in the National Weight Control Registry (NWCR) and those who live in Colorado have reasons for being active that are connected to their personal values and go far beyond hoping to reach a certain number on the scale. Many have told us that exercise gives them a sense of purpose and a way to forge connections between their minds and their bodies. They have linked their daily activity to other things in their lives that are important to them. For example, some of them view their workouts as a time for meditation or prayer. Others organize and plan their day as they exercise. Many have built movement into their social routine so that it forms an essential part of their relationships with the people they value most.

// *How* will you find the time?

We all live fast-paced lives, and most of us are constantly time challenged. It's likely that physical activity will have to displace some other activities you are currently doing. What can you do without in order to fit in fitness? Perhaps there's a TV show you'd be willing to skip—or you can make the decision to watch it while you're exercising. Or maybe you can get up an hour earlier in the morning.

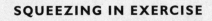

SQUEEZING IN EXERCISE

Even if your schedule is jam-packed, you may be able to slot in your activity simply by making inactive time active. How? Anytime you're sitting down, ask yourself: "Is there any way I could be moving while doing this same activity?"

IF YOU'RE . . .	TRY THIS
Watching TV	Walk on a treadmill or use an exercise bike
Watching your child's soccer practice	Walk laps around the field
Getting together with a friend	Go for a walk instead of going out to eat (or save the meal for after the walk)
Having a meeting with a colleague	Hold a walking meeting—go for a stroll outside
Talking on the phone	Make it a rule to stand or pace when talking on the phone

Remember, what you're really committing to is losing weight once and for all. Don't just start this program and hope it will work out—think through your day and consider where you'll find time for movement.

By the time you reach phase 3 of the Colorado Diet, you'll be devoting 70 minutes a day to physical activity. Sounds like a lot, but consider this: Seventy minutes is less than 5 percent of your day. In those few minutes, you can fix your metabolism and lose weight forever. Think of it that way, and it sounds like a great deal!

// *What* type of exercise would you enjoy?

Many people tell us that they just don't like exercise. It would be pretty depressing if you started this program thinking you had to do something you dislike for the rest of your life. Changing your perspective comes down to changing your attitude. Those slender Coloradans and the people in the NWCR don't view physical activity as something they *must* do but rather as something they're *eager* to do. People in our clinic who focus on the benefits they get from moving their bodies have an easier time sticking to their activity plans than those who view exercise as a chore forced on them. Convince yourself that you won't enjoy being active and you won't. And you're likely to quit before you've reaped the rewards. If you eagerly anticipate how much better you'll feel after a workout—and when you're able to maintain a healthy weight—you'll put yourself on the road to success. There's a lot to look forward to. Being active and fit lifts your mood, helps you sleep better, and boosts your energy. It improves your memory and may even ward off cognitive decline as you age.

By following our advice, you'll find a type of movement that you like—or at least one that you don't dislike. This can be as simple as walking, but it could also be taking an exercise class, riding a bike, or joining a volleyball team. Along the way, we'll show you how to seek out others who enjoy living a healthy lifestyle.

That being said, make sure you have realistic expectations about how physical activity will affect you. You may be moving muscles that haven't been used in a while, and you might feel tired or a little sore after activity. At the same time, though, following through on your committment to exercise can bring a sense of accomplishment. Try to concentrate on the positives. If you don't experience any at first, know that you will soon enough. Trust us, after a few sessions, exercise *will* start to feel good. As you get more physically fit and lose weight, you'll find it much easier to move your body, and you'll feel energized, not pooped, after exercise. By starting slowly and increasing your movement in small steps, we'll help you minimize the bad feelings and maximize the good ones.

// *What*, when, where, and with whom?

It's not enough just to say you'll become active and develop a Colorado Mind-Set. You have to work out the details. Plan for adding exercise into your day just as you would plan for a family trip to Disney World. Decide how you'll organize your day to fit in all the important things—and movement is important.

First up: What will you do? Beginning on page 72, we explain that you have two different options for increasing your activity—the Structured Plan and the Flexible Plan—but no matter which one you choose, you still must decide *exactly* what you'll do. This will take effort and planning.

Next, consider when and where you'll work out. On Sundays, designate a time for exercise for the upcoming week. It doesn't have to be the same hour every day, but remember that habits, routines, and rituals conserve willpower. You might be someone who prefers to exercise solo because you view your workout as "me" time or you don't want to depend on someone else's schedule. Or you may find it helpful to get a friend or family member to be active with you—a walking partner or a tennis partner, for instance. Some people like to be part of groups; if that's you, join clubs or teams or enroll in exercise classes. And still others like to mix it up! There are so many options. Experiment and see which one works best for you.

// *Where* can you find social support?

Research shows that you'll be more successful in making behavior changes if the people around you back your efforts and if you feel accountable. Because incorporating exercise does disrupt your routine at first, it's especially helpful to find people to support you—by cheering you on or by simply not giving you a hard time when you can't join them for an outing because you've got a workout scheduled. Spouses, family members, neighbors, friends, coworkers, even your doctor can all potentially be part of you've got a team. Because the people who support you are usually the important people in your life, they'll be with you during the rough times, and you won't want to let them down. Two exceptionally smart ideas: Find a partner to go on the Colorado Diet with you so you can motivate each other, and/or use your Facebook page as a tool—post your physical activity goals and ask your friends to provide you with support and encouragement. Hiring a personal trainer or signing up for a series of exercise classes can also increase your accountability. There are even Web sites that give you online access to an accountability program. Some of these sites provide a way for friends to add comments; others may give you a financial incentive to achieve your goals.

GETTING STARTED

On the Colorado Diet, you choose between two activity plans. Both approaches are equally effective. What's key is that you pick the one that's most likely to work for you over the next 4 months as you develop your Mile-High Metabolism and lose weight. After that, you can alternate between the two approaches, if you'd like.

Your two options are the Structured Plan and the Flexible Plan. On the Structured Plan, you work up to 70 minutes of planned activity 6 days a week. On the Flexible Plan, you'll eventually be doing 35 minutes of planned activity 6 days a week combined with moving more in your daily life and measuring your lifestyle activity with a pedometer. Both plans include a rest day. Don't worry—we explain exactly how to get there, step-by-step, in each phase of the Colorado Diet.

Planned activity is exactly what it sounds like—physical activity that you schedule in advance. It can be walking oudoors, biking, playing tennis, walking on a treadmill, taking an aerobics class, or any number of other ways to move your body. Just be sure to do *something* each day. You can mix and match different activities on different days, but our experience suggests that the more routine you make it—such as playing tennis every Tuesday and Thursday and walking with a neighbor on Mondays and Wednesdays—the more likely you'll be to follow through. Be realistic: There's no sense in designating a cardio class as your planned activity if the class times don't mesh with your schedule. And pick something appealing. If it's not fun, you probably won't stick with it. For more information on choosing a planned activity, see "Finding Your Perfect Fit" on page 74.

MAKING EXERCISE WORK

Don is one of our patients who lost 42 pounds and kept it off. He had no trouble changing his diet, but he struggled to get in his 70 minutes of physical activity. He first tried exercising in the middle of the day, then during late afternoon, but work issues constantly interfered with his workout. Finally, Don realized that he was always free early in the morning and decided he'd exercise at 6:00 a.m. It was hard at first, but he gradually developed a routine of getting up a little earlier and going to the fitness center. To make it easier, he decided to set his alarm for 5:00 a.m. and dress for the gym as soon as he got up. He packed a bag every night with office clothes. After his workout, he'd shower and shave and head for the office. He was surprised to find that after a few months, this routine was effortless. He even made some new friends among the early-morning crowd at the fitness center. And he loved how good he felt knowing he'd gotten exercise out of the way.

Lifestyle activity forms the foundation of the Flexible Plan. Just getting through your day requires *some* motion—walking from your car to the house, climbing stairs, navigating the grocery store, chasing your child around the house. Unfortunately, we often strive to avoid or minimize any movement. We look for the closest parking space. We take the elevator to our office. Many of us sit in front of a computer most of our workday. Our lives are set up in such a way that we don't need to move much at all.

People in our clinic are amazed by how much they can increase lifestyle physical activity with some simple strategies. Our research

(continued on page 76)

FINDING YOUR PERFECT FIT

Here are some things to consider as you choose a planned activity. What types of activity did you enjoy in your younger days? Did you play tennis or golf or soccer? Did you like swimming or dancing? Are you drawn to team sports, or do you prefer individual sports? Do you belong to a gym or health club, or would you like to join one?

Answering these questions can help you pinpoint activities to try first. If your initial choice isn't a home run, select something else—but be sure to allow enough time for your body to adjust to a new activity before crossing it off your list.

Not sure where to begin? You might start with walking. Many people don't consider walking *real* exercise—and that can be a pro or a con. If you don't consider it "exercise," you might be more inclined to do it. Conversely, you may not think it's going to do you any good, so you don't prioritize it. Let us be clear: Walking is both easy and effective. It is the most frequently performed activity by participants in the NWCR, and its health benefits are numerous and well established. Research studies have shown that walking helps prevent heart disease, diabetes, and cancer. A study from Duke University found that walking 30 minutes a day greatly reduced the chances of developing metabolic syndrome—a group of risk factors that occur together and increase the risk of coronary artery disease, stroke, and type 2 diabetes.

To start, simply walk at a pace that is comfortable for you—starting out at 2 miles per hour is perfectly okay. You can pick up the pace to 3 to 4 miles per hour (a mile every 15 to 20 minutes) as you get more fit. You might want to engage your friends or coworkers and starting a walking group.

If you're still not sure what activity you'd like, make a game of it. Test a few different planned activities and see which ones you enjoy. You could be surprised by what you discover.

Types of Planned Physical Activity

Aerobics or fitness classes	Skating
Basketball	Skiing
Cycling outdoors or on a stationary bike	Soccer
	Spinning
Dancing	Stair climbing or using step machines
Elliptical machines	
Golf	Swimming
Hiking	Tennis
Pilates	Volleyball
Playing Wii Fit	Walking outdoors or on a treadmill
Running	Yoga
Running in place	Zumba

shows that the average American adult takes about 5,500 steps per day and that most people can easily increase that to 7,000 or 7,500 steps daily. Just look for ways to move more (see the ideas in Lifestyle Activities on the opposite page), and measure your lifestyle physical activity with a pedometer to accurately count the steps you take. For instance, if you arrive 5 minutes early to a meeting, walk up and down the hall instead of sitting to wait for the others—that may add several hundred steps. Your ultimate goal is to get 7,000 steps a day, and you'll supplement that with 35 minutes of planned activity.

Most people find it useful to check their pedometers every few hours and adjust their movement to ensure that they fit in their 7,000 steps by the end of the day. An easy rule of thumb: Five minutes of walking equates to approximately 500 steps.

It helps to be attentive to your usual activity patterns. For example, you may see that your Tuesdays and Saturdays are active and you have no trouble hitting your goal, but Mondays and Thursdays are more sedentary, and you need to come up with strategies to meet your step goal on those days.

Make a habit of checking the pedometer regularly and you'll be more likely to stay on track. It's easier to add a few hundred steps here and there throughout the day than to squeeze in thousands of steps at night.

// *Picking* Your Plan

How do you decide between the two exercise plans? It doesn't matter which one you select. They both lead to a Mile-High Metabolism.

CHOOSE THE STRUCTURED PLAN if you won't remember to clip on

LIFESTYLE ACTIVITIES

It's not difficult to work extra movement into your typical day. Here are just a few ideas. You'll find plenty more at America On the Move (americaonthemove.org), a national nonprofit initiative we started several years ago to translate our science of small changes into ways to help people move more and eat better.

- Don't look for the closest parking spot—look for the one farthest from your destination.
- Get off the bus one stop early.
- Use a bathroom on a different floor.
- Go the long way when walking to a meeting.
- Walk around the block when picking up the mail.
- Do an extra lap around the grocery store.
- Take the stairs for one floor up or two floors down.
- Walk and talk when on the phone.
- Walk whenever a commercial comes on TV.
- Print documents at a distant printer.
- Walk to a neighbor's house instead of calling on the phone.

your pedometer every day or if you don't like the idea of wearing one. Some people prefer to focus on exercise once a day so that it's done and over with; the structured approach works best for them. This plan is also the better option if your job doesn't give you the freedom to increase your movement.

PURCHASING A PEDOMETER

If you decide to follow the Flexible Plan, you'll need a pedometer to keep on track. This small device is usually worn on your belt or waistband (like a small pager) and counts and displays the number of steps you take. It provides powerful and immediate feedback about where you are in relation to your daily step goal.

You don't have to spend a lot of money to get a good pedometer; they run $15 to $20. We prefer ones that simply measure the number of steps you take (that's really all you need), but there are pedometers that estimate how many calories you're using, too.

When you find a pedometer, test it. Walk and count out 50 steps; if the display says 40 to 60 steps, it's doing its job. If it records fewer than 40 steps or more than 60, the device needs to be readjusted or repositioned on your waist. No waistband on your clothes? Try placing the pedometer on your ankle or neckline, and again check it for accuracy. If a pedometer worn at your waist or another location doesn't seem to do a good job measuring your steps, consider pedometers that can count steps when carried in a pocket or purse. They are more expensive but may be worthwhile if you have a body type or walking style that does not work well with traditional pedometers. Finally, there are many other devices on the market today—such as wireless trackers like the Fitbit clip-on plus armbands and activity bracelets—that count steps as well as track minutes of activity. They are more expensive. While they're not necessary for your success, you might find them helpful in achieving your goals.

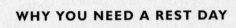

WHY YOU NEED A REST DAY

Building and maintaining your new lifestyle requires that you periodically give your body time to rest and recover. Even professional athletes don't work hard every day. We recommend you take a day off once a week, whether you're on the structured or the flexible activity plan. Just like sleep renews your mind every 24 hours and resets your willpower and metabolism for the next day, a day off from planned activity every 7 days gives your muscles the opportunity to repair themselves and get ready for the next week of activity. This is especially important if you are new to activity or are increasing the amount you normally do. You may be sore and a rest and recovery day will help you hit the next week with more energy as well as prevent injuries. We also believe having one day off a week is good for your mind-set. Use it as a day to reflect and enjoy your accomplishments over the last week.

SELECT THE FLEXIBLE PLAN if you can't allocate extended periods of time for activity or if you prefer small bursts of activity instead of longer ones. This plan may also be better for you if your lifestyle is fairly active or offers multiple opportunities to move more throughout the day.

Before you decide, you might clip on a pedometer and measure how much activity you get in an average day (see "Purchasing a Pedometer" on the opposite page). It's probably less than you think. Take the case of John, one of our patients. He's a business executive who leads a typically busy, productive life. His to-do list is long, and his life is full of work, family, and social obligations. When we asked him to rate his level of lifestyle activity, he was sure that it was high, because he was always on the go. He guessed that he must be taking at least 7,000 steps per day, maybe more. But when John started using a pedometer, he was shocked to discover that he was averaging only about 4,000 steps daily. Our brains tend to register stress and busyness as activity, but as John found out, this doesn't necessarily equate to physical movement.

EXCUSE-PROOF YOUR WORKOUT

Most people don't have trouble upping their daily lifestyle activity, but they do face obstacles regarding planned activity. Choosing the best exercise approach for you, and tailoring it to your schedule, helps you overcome the barriers, as does reminding yourself of your purpose and making exercise a habit, routine, or ritual. Once you get going with physical activity, you'll want to keep moving simply because you'll feel toned, strong, healthy, and energetic. But if you haven't felt that way in a while, this can be a hard statement to believe! That's one reason we hear the same objections to exercise again and again in our clinic. Here are the solutions we give to our patients for the most common obstacles.

// *Excuse:* I have no time.

SOLUTION: Prioritize activity by tying it directly to other things that are important to you. And redefine what's important. For

HOLLY'S TIPS

Prioritizing Exercise

I often work with our patients on daily priorities. When I explain how much physical activity they need to "fix" their metabolisms, they're often disappointed. They say, "I just don't have the time" or "My knees won't take it." Some will even whip out their calendars and show me *exactly* how busy they are. They just don't see how they can possibly find another 70 minutes in their day. Well, the truth of the matter is, we all find time for things in our lives that are our priorities. Sometimes, I ask my patients if they could incorporate regular physical activity into their lives if they knew they would win a $100 million lottery or if moving their bodies would somehow find a cure for cancer or prevent a child from going hungry. The answer is always yes. People with bad knees would head for the pool or try other non-weight-bearing alternatives. Busy people would suddenly find the time. No matter what you have going on in your life, you can always carve minutes for the things most important to you, and what could be more important than the health and well-being you'll gain by exercising?

instance, how much TV do you watch? Would you give up one show? If you don't want to give up TV time, then find a way to multitask. Put a treadmill in front of the screen and walk your way through your favorite program. Remember, too, that you don't have to complete your planned activity all at once. It's okay to spend 15 minutes before breakfast, at lunch, and before bedtime.

// *Excuse:* I'm too tired.

SOLUTION: Get moving anyway. You'll discover that physical activity actually boosts your energy. Most of the time, just getting moving is the biggest hurdle. Tell yourself, "I'm just going to do it for 10 minutes, and if I'm still too tired, I can stop." After 10 minutes, you'll probably feel able to handle 10 more. If this doesn't work, move your activity time to the morning, when your willpower is strongest. (You may need to go to bed earlier to adopt this approach.) Try this morning routine for 2 weeks and see if you find it easier.

// *Excuse:* It hurts.

SOLUTION: Find something that doesn't. No matter what your ailment and no matter how out of shape you may be, there's *something* you can do without pain. If walking strains your knees, try an exercise bike. If that's painful, too, try exercising in the pool. Still not having luck? Consult a trainer or physical therapist for advice. Don't give up—you have the power to figure this out!

// *Excuse:* I have no place to do it.

SOLUTION: Walk—you can do that anywhere. If all else fails, you can walk laps around your living room or the local mall. Get creative. Break down your day into increments from the moment you get up until bedtime. How could you move more throughout the day? Walk whenever you are on your cell phone (and it's safe to do so), or find a track that's on your way home from work. If you prefer to walk with others, join a walking group or simply grab a friend and get moving.

// *Excuse:* It's too hot, too cold, too snowy, too humid, too rainy—too something.

SOLUTION: Head inside. Join a gym. Put a stationary bike in front of your TV. Walk laps around the local mall or a large retail store. Climb stairs in an indoor building. Try a DVD or an exercise tape. Find a friend with an exercise bike or a treadmill and ask if you can come over and use it. Come up with your own "last resort" exercise plan.

// *Excuse:* I hate exercise.

SOLUTION: Do an attitude adjustment. Write down what you like about exercise—even if it is just one thing and even if that thing is that you like how you feel when it's over! You can also focus on the good things that will happen as a result of exercising. For example, you'll have more energy, sleep better, get a mood boost—the list can go on and on. Try some positive reinforcement: Consider it play. If you believe it will feel good, it will. Revisit your purpose and again see if you can tie why you want to lose weight to your activity routine. Or try salsa dancing, tai chi, or something else that doesn't feel like exercise. Any activity counts!

———

Ease into it. We don't expect that you will necessarily love working out right from the get-go. Our research using a small-changes approach taught us that most people are better at making gradual improvements than big ones. This is especially true for physical activity, where giving people pedometers and small goals for increasing steps has led to greater increases in physical activity than giving them a goal of 30 minutes a day of physical activity. If it's been years since you exercised regularly, you may be a little creaky at first, and your muscles may ache. But these problems will disappear as you grow accustomed to our fitness plan. In the meantime, start slowly and give yourself time to adjust. As your fitness level improves, exercise will feel much easier and more pleasurable.

Prepare to Eat Smarter:
Dining the Colorado Diet Way

CHAPTER 5

THE LOGIC BEHIND THE Colorado Diet is really quite simple and is based on the science we described in earlier chapters. Over 16 weeks, we'll help you fix your metabolism so it works the way it was meant to. At each phase of the plan, we give you diet parameters that are matched to the state of your metabolism, increasing your body's ability to burn fat so you lose weight. At the end, you'll have a Mile-High Metabolism and know how to eat smarter to provide the best fuel for your restored metabolism. And you won't be facing a life of deprivation—you'll be able to eat the way your healthy, active friends do.

Most of you are probably starting with an inflexible metabolism. So that you can lose weight with an inflexible metabolism, we initially restrict what you eat to the foods that promote fat loss. As your metabolism gets more flexible, we'll add more types of foods to the menu. In phase 3 of the Colorado Diet, we'll teach you to eat smarter so that you provide your body with the best fuel for a robust metabolism. You'll be pleasantly surprised at both the amount and variety of food you can eat as part of your well-rounded diet. Healthy eating is fun when you have a healthy metabolism to match.

The two of us have conducted numerous studies examining just about every major diet out there. We know that most people seeking weight loss expect something radical—no fat or no sugar or low carbs—that suddenly makes life wonderful. If there were such a diet, we would have discovered it by now. Our research shows that many people are able to lose weight on radical diets but very few are able to maintain those eating plans for long. Over and over, we see that once you attain a Mile-High Metabolism, a reasonable, varied diet is what works. It may not be sexy, but it's the way active, healthy people eat—and you can eat this way, too. By following just a few simple guidelines, you'll be surprised at how easy it is to lose weight and achieve a Mile-High Metabolism so you can maintain that loss.

So there's no magic combination of foods for maintaining a healthy weight. But there are some common factors. Participants in the National Weight Control Registry, competitive athletes, and healthy people in Colorado tend to eat diets high in protein and carbo-hydrate (but the right kinds of carbs) and low in fat. They eat high-fat and high-sugar foods as treats—not as everyday foods. They get very few calories from beverages, and they watch their portion sizes. They don't frequent all-you-can-eat buffets. In other words, they eat smart, but they don't worry constantly about restricting their calories. A big reason is because their active lifestyles and flexible metabolisms burn a lot of calories.

EATING THE RIGHT FOODS AT THE RIGHT TIME

You don't need to count calories on the Colorado Diet because we've made it easy to choose the right combination of foods for the various states your metabolism is in. Based on what we know about the body's natural priority system for using nutrients— protein, carbohydrate, and fat—and how the state of your metabolism affects that, we give you diet parameters in each phase that maximize fat-burning and minimize fat storage. But even the healthiest foods can be overeaten, so you do need to pay close attention to portion sizes.

One question we're often asked is whether all calories are equal, or whether some calories are more fattening than others. This has been a focus of our research for many years, and the answer is: "It depends." So many things affect the way an individual's body uses calories—your total energy intake, your physical activity level, your body size. In general, though, your body can use protein, carbohydrate, and fat as fuel, but it prefers to use them in a specific order.

Protein is your metabolism's first choice. The protein in food is broken down into its individual components, called amino acids. Some of these are used for your body's housekeeping functions (maintaining muscle, making hormones, and general cell repair), but all the rest is burned. The fact that the body doesn't have anywhere to store excess protein is probably why you fill up on protein faster than you do on carbs or fats. Eating it gives you built-in appetite and calorie control. Think about it. You probably could eat a quart of ice cream (mostly sugar and fat) if you tried but would struggle to wolf down an equivalent amount of lean meat, poultry, or fish. We recommend a lot of lean protein in the early phases of the Colorado Diet because we know it's satiating and it will all be burned.

Carbohydrates are the next in line. A little bit of the carbohydrate you eat is used to replenish the glycogen stores in your muscles or liver. (Glycogen is a form of carbohydrate that muscles use for fuel.) Your body only rarely converts excess carbohydrate (or protein, for that matter) into fat. Research conducted by Dr. Eric Jéquier at the University of Lausanne has shown that you must eat about 1,000 extra carb calories a day above your energy needs for a week before your body begins to turn carbs into fat. Your muscles like having carbohydrates around because they provide quick energy. This is probably because early in mankind's history, protein was hard to come by in the diet, and people were lucky to get the minimal amount needed to sustain their body systems. By contrast, carbs have always been abundant in the human diet, and the body has come to rely on them as the primary source of fuel. That's why athletes "carbo-load" before long endurance events.

Your body turns to fat-burning only after it has depleted all of its protein and carbohydrate. While your body can't store protein or carbs very efficiently, it has a virtually unlimited capacity to store fat. The amount of fat you burn is the difference between how much energy your body needs and how much energy you take in from protein and carbohydrate. For example, several years ago Jim did a study where he had people follow a high-carbohydrate diet for 2 weeks and then a high-fat diet for 2 weeks. Both diets supplied 50 percent more calories than the study participants needed to maintain their body weight. He found that most of the excess energy was stored regardless of the diet composition, although a higher proportion of the excess was stored on the high-fat diet. This makes sense from a fuel hierarchy view. If you consume extra carbs, you will burn more carbs but will need to tap into fewer stored fat calories. If you eat excess fat, it goes into your fat cells and, since it's not needed for energy, will stay there.

Most fat-burning occurs between meals. After a meal, your body primarily uses the protein and carbohydrate in the meal and puts the fat into your fat cells. Between meals, when the carbohydrate has been depleted and insulin levels are low, your body draws on the stored fat and converts it to fuel for your muscles. You burn less fat when your total energy needs are low and met mostly with protein and carbohydrate—or if you eat another large meal before you have used up all your protein and carbohydrate from the previous meal. We limit fat during the early phases of the Colorado Diet to force your body to use stored fat for fuel. We specifically limit saturated fat (in full-fat dairy products, fatty meats, and butter), since studies show that it tends to be stored more readily than unsaturated fat (olive oil, avocado, nuts, canola oil). Saturated fat is also associated with an increased risk of heart disease.

What this means is that your body stores fat when you overeat regardless of whether the excess calories come from protein, carbohydrate, or fat. That's because when you eat any form of calories in excess, it prevents your metabolism from burning the fat stores you've already accumulated. If you take in too much protein or carbohydrate, the fat that you would have burned if you didn't overeat will be stored as body fat. When you eat excess fat, it prevents your body from burning the fat you already have and instead stores it in your fat cells.

GETTING RID OF BODY FAT

To lose weight, you have to eliminate some of the fat you have stored in your body. So how do you achieve this? You can do it just by eating less. But a better way is also to up your physical activity level. You can also tweak your diet so you burn more fat. Most diets do this by restricting your food intake. This works, because if you take in fewer calories than you use, your body has to dig into your fat stores to make up the difference. The problem is that most people can't live on tiny portions indefinitely, so this strategy isn't sustainable for the long haul. Even if you stick to a low-cal diet, you probably won't keep the weight off, because as you eat less, your metabolism slows down so that you need fewer calories. As soon as you stop the food restriction, you start storing fat very quickly. A better way to get your body to draw down on its fat reserves is to not feed it foods that are easy to store as fat and feed it foods that promote fat-burning instead.

Foods that are low in energy density fit the bill. Energy density, a concept pioneered by Dr. Barbara Rolls at Pennsylvania State University, is a measure of how many calories a food has for its given volume. Research done by Dr. Rolls has shown that the satisfaction factor delivered by a food is directly related to its volume. Foods with lots of bulk and water (such as broccoli, spinach, and cucumbers) have a low energy density—their calorie count is modest even for large serving sizes. Foods high in sugar and fat (like candy, chips, and cookies) have a high energy density—they pack lots of calories into a tiny portion. For instance, for the 224 calories in a small order of fast-food fries, you could have one large head (23 ounces) of broccoli.

We want you to get in the habit of choosing foods with a low energy density. Foods high in fat are usually very energy-dense, and simple carbohydrates (like sugar) have a higher energy density than more complex carbohydrates, such as vegetables, that are naturally packaged with water and fiber. In the early phases of the Colorado Diet, we limit the amount of fat you get, and we limit you to carbohydrates with a very low energy density. These carbs allow you to reduce the number of calories you eat so you force your body to use its stored fat for fuel.

THE THREE PHASES OF THE COLORADO DIET

A Mile-High Metabolism can only be created in stages. That's why we've broken the process down. Each phase is matched to the state of your metabolism. They're specifically designed to promote weight loss while fixing your metabolism and integrating what you eat with how you move.

Looking back to our bathtub metaphor, your objective in phase 1, **Reignite,** is to limit the water coming into your tub as you work to unclog your bathtub drain. In just 2 weeks, you'll turn on your fat-burning engine and experience rapid weight loss—you can expect to lose 8 to 10 pounds in phase 1. Refined carbohydrates (white flour and sugar) and too much fat trigger cravings, are easy to overeat, and promote fat storage. In fact, when you have a broken metabolism, even some healthy carbs—such as whole grains and beans—can slow fat-burning and prevent weight loss. That's why phase 1 is very high in lean protein and restricts certain carbohydrates and fats. You will eat veggies and other foods that keep you full without lots of calories. In this phase, we emphasize vegetables as your primary carb source, because they're loaded with vitamins, minerals, and other nutrients that keep your immune system strong, maintain your bones and muscles, and support the energetic and active lifestyle you're developing. We also gradually introduce you to physical activity in this phase.

Phase 2, **Rebuild,** lasts 6 weeks. You ramp up your physical activity in this phase, eventually reaching 70 minutes a day, and that increases the amount of energy your body needs. This phase is critical for everyone but is especially important for the aging gainers we described in Chapter 2, whose metabolisms have slowly decreased over time. Your muscles become more sensitive to insulin, create more mitochondria (the energy centers of cells), and get better at burning fat. Here you'll add some foods to your diet that have a little more fat along with a little carbohydrate and a very small amount of foods (like fruit) whose energy comes mainly from simple sugars; the additional carbs help fuel your increased activity. This acclimates your body to using what you eat and allows fat-burning to occur throughout the day. Active muscles need a lot of carbohydrate for fuel, but they also tap into some fat during exercise. On recovery days, when you take a break from exercise, your muscles will repair and replenish themselves, and your increasingly flexible metabolism will burn mostly carbs after meals and mostly fat in between them. And because your metabolism is working so well, you're allowed an indulgence meal every week—an opportunity to eat whatever you want. You'll continue to lose weight during this phase, typically at a rate of 1 to 2 pounds per week.

By the time you enter phase 3, **Reinforce,** you'll be well on your way to a Mile-High Metabolism, but you still need to nurture it. You have more leeway in your diet because all that physical activity you're doing acts as a buffer to limit the impact of any one meal on fat-burning or body weight. During this phase, you can add more protein and fat options to your diet as well as significantly more carbohydrates and sugar-containing fruits, because your body has now been trained to burn them. This is the phase during which the easy gainers described in Chapter 2 will really notice a difference. For the first time, they may realize that it's possible to stay slim even if they don't always eat "perfectly." Their bodies are now primed to adjust to the occasional treat.

At this point, you are doing 70 minutes per day of physical activity, and you need to ensure you are eating adequate carbohydrates to fuel this level of activity. You'll still be losing weight during this phase, typically at a rate of up to 1 to 2 pounds per week. You get to add two indulgence meals per week, in which you can eat anything you want. By the time they finish this phase, many of our patients say they feel like they've reinvented themselves. Use this phase to solidify your new habits so you are prepared to live as an active, fit, healthy person now and in the future. After these 8 weeks, you'll be ready to move on to the maintenance phase, as we discuss in Chapter 9.

HOW TO FOLLOW THE COLORADO DIET

Our plan calls for six meals each day (three meals, three snacks) to provide a steady supply of energy for daily activities and lots of protein to preserve lean body mass and build your stamina for physical activity.

For each phase, you'll choose from three categories of foods for your meals and snacks: proteins, carbohydrates, and fats. We provide a list of foods for each category and tell you what the portion size needs to be. The categories are:

THE LEANEST PROTEINS. Protein is a critical part of every phase because it's the body's top fuel choice and because, calorie for calorie, it's more filling than carbohydrate or fat. But some protein comes with fat. For instance, bacon and sausage are high in protein but also derive close to 80 percent of their calories from fat. Cheese, while a good source of protein and calcium, is also very high in fat, generally over 50 percent of calories. We start you off with the very leanest proteins in phase 1. As you progress, you'll be able to eat protein that comes packaged with some fat. However, lean protein should be your predominant choice through all three phases.

Protein is particularly important in the mornings. A recent study from the University of Kansas revealed that people felt much fuller during the day when their weight-loss diets included more protein at breakfast. Our work with NWCR participants and successful weight-loss patients has also found that eating protein with breakfast helps people manage their hunger better throughout the day.

CARBOHYDRATES. Carbohydrates can range from simple sugars to vegetables to foods containing whole grains. You are permitted to have different types of carbs in different phases. The carb categories are called *Reignite* carbs, *Rebuild* carbs, *Reinforce* carbs, and vegetable carbs. We give you a simple rule for when and how much to choose from each list for your daily meals. Reignite carbs are difficult to either overeat or store as fat. They are always your go-to carbs when you see the number on the scale starting to creep up. The carbs in the Rebuild and Reinforce phases are good sources of fuel for physical activity. Active muscles have a much higher need for carbohydrate as fuel than sedentary muscles do. Vegetable carbohydrates have a very low energy density and can be eaten without restriction on all phases of the Colorado Diet. As you become more active during these later phases, you'll be able to add more carbs— even, on occasion, some that are rich in simple sugar. Your new metabolism will be able to handle them.

ONLY THE HEALTHIEST FATS. Your body needs some dietary fat to keep the membranes of your cells functioning so that nutrients and other substances can easily enter your cells. But you need much less than you're eating now. The fats you'll eat during phase 1 are essential fats, the ones your body can't make on its own and the ones least likely to up your risk of heart disease and other health problems. The amount of fat is limited so that you don't contribute to your body fat stores. As you increase your capacity to burn rather than store fat, we'll expand the types of fats you can eat.

Unsaturated fats, like the ones that come from plants (olive oil, canola oil) or fish (fish oil) are the healthiest. Avoid saturated and trans fats. Trans fats are often used to extend the shelf life of processed foods. Limit them as much as possible, because they have been shown to contribute to heart disease. Want a shortcut to figuring out if a fat is healthy? Take a look at it at room temperature. Healthy fats like olive oil are liquid at room temperature, and these liquid fats are the ones least likely to clog your drain (or your arteries).

LEARNING TO BE FLEXIBLE

Lisa never had a weight problem until she started working for a nonprofit company that required her to travel 3 days a week. Before then, she was able to eat most things in moderation. She loves her new work, but her change in lifestyle brought unwanted weight gain. Over the last 10 years, she put on about 30 pounds. The weight gain was gradual, and she didn't notice it much from year to year. When she turned 52, though, she suddenly decided she needed to do something. She came to our clinic because she felt drained of energy all the time. She was tired of lugging around the extra body fat. She just couldn't keep the weight off the way she could when she was younger. She admitted it was harder to make healthy food choices on the road, and her weekly tennis matches and regular practice had to take a backseat to her travel schedule.

Lisa's story is common. Her metabolism had become inflexible over the years—in part because she was getting older (see the aging gainer example in Chapter 2) and in part because her activity level had dropped below the point where her body could adjust to the food she ate. Lisa agreed to try the Colorado Diet and lost

THE COLORADO DIET RULES

You'll follow five diet rules in every phase of the Colorado Diet. The first two are always the same. The specifics of the remaining three vary from phase to phase (we'll remind you of the rules and spell them out in each chapter).

10 pounds in phase 1 even though she was on the road 3 days a week. She was ecstatic. She says: "I'm not going to lie, the first 2 weeks were strict. But after 2 days, I actually felt better and now am working on increasing my activity in phase 2 so I can get back the metabolism I had when I was younger and eat some of the foods I love." She was able to find ways to stick to the plan despite her travel schedule. For example, she carried individual packets of orange-flavored Crystal Light in her purse to stir into nonfat Greek yogurt (she said it tastes like orange sherbet), and she made a habit of ordering an egg-white omelet or oatmeal through room service the night before. Making a healthy breakfast a no-brainer helped her resist the temptation of the high-fat convenience foods she used to rely on.

Lisa is progressing through phase 2 and gradually adding in her Rebuild carbohydrates. She is down 15 pounds and still losing. She wants to drop another 15 pounds and is figuring out how to add in her activity both at home and on the road. She has built in a routine for each that works for her. Her mind-set is positive. She believes she has found a way to get back to the place she was 15 years ago, and she feels empowered to live her new lifestyle.

1. **EAT SIX TIMES A DAY.** Your meals should be spaced every 2 to 4 hours to keep your insulin levels stable, to help you manage your hunger, and to maintain your energy levels.

2. **HAVE BREAKFAST WITHIN AN HOUR OF WAKING UP.** Eating breakfast is a harbinger of weight-loss success. It's a

habit the majority of individuals in the National Weight Control Registry follow, and several research studies show that people who eat breakfast weigh less than those who don't. Researchers think this is because the morning meal helps you manage your hunger better during the day and results in an overall lower daily energy intake. We recommend eating within an hour of getting up because we've found that people who wait longer than this are more likely to skip breakfast and use this as an excuse to overeat later in the day.

3. **DON'T COUNT CALORIES, MEASURE PORTIONS.** With the Colorado Diet, you don't have to monitor every calorie you put into your mouth. If you stick to the recommended portion sizes, you'll create a negative energy deficit while minimizing your hunger. One problem with calorie counting is that most people aren't very good at it. Many research studies have shown that people tend to dramatically underestimate the amount of food they eat (interestingly, people also tend to overestimate how much physical activity they get). Accurately remembering what you eat is not easy. In fact, one of Jim's research studies revealed that even experienced dietitians underestimate their food intake. Portion sizing takes food amnesia out of the question, provided you measure, not guess—at least at first. You have to become very familiar with what a portion of different foods looks like before you can eyeball a tablespoon of olive oil drizzled on some greens or a

6-ounce chicken breast, and some people never really get it right.

4. **HAVE THE RiGHT CARB AND PROTEIN MIX AT EVERY MEAL.** Pick one option from the carb list for the phase you're in and one from the Leanest Proteins list. For at least three of your meals, you should choose vegetables as your only carbohydrate source. We list these vegetables in the charts in every phase. You can have as much of these as you'd like, and you can mix and match them at a meal. For example, you can have asparagus with a drizzle of lemon juice and a large salad with lettuce, tomatoes, carrots, and celery at the same meal. For the other three meals, you can choose any phase-appropriate carbohydrate (for instance, fat-free milk, oatmeal, or pumpkin in phase 1). If you desire, you can also have some veggies in combination with the other carbohydrates for these three meals.

5. **EAT A HEALTHY FAT TWICE A DAY.** If fat is most easily stored as body fat, why not cut it out completely? Two reasons. You actually need some fat for your metabolism to perform optimally. Second, people like fat—we're used to eating it, and it makes our diets more satisfying. But you need only a tiny amount for your body to function well and to make your diet more interesting. We've done a lot of research showing that fat is the nutrient most likely to be overconsumed. In one of our studies, when we increased the fat content of people's diets, they spontaneously increased the total number of calories they ate without realizing it. Your fat options widen as you

progress through the phases, but we always emphasize unsaturated fats, because they're the least likely to clog your arteries or be stored as body fat.

Are you ready to unclog your drain and keep the water flowing freely for good? Let's get started!

Reignite Your Metabolism

The Colorado Diet Phase 1
(Weeks 1–2)

CHAPTER 6

IF WE'VE DONE OUR JOB, you understand why you need to fix both your diet and your metabolism to be successful in losing weight *and* keeping it off. Hopefully you're on board and thinking, "I can do this. I want to do this." But you're probably asking yourself, "Where do I start?"

Right here. This 2-week phase is carefully designed to help you lose weight while beginning to shift your body out of fat-storing mode and into fat-burning mode. We like to say it reignites your fat burners while producing a rapid weight loss. When patients come to us and say, "I'm doing everything right and the scale just won't budge," we put them on phase 1 of the Colorado Diet. It has *never* failed to produce results. You'll lose weight very quickly—most people drop at least 8 to 10 pounds in phase 1—and that keeps you energized and motivated while you're unclogging your drain.

PHASE I GOALS

- Lose weight by eating foods that won't be stored as fat

- Begin to fix your metabolism by establishing physical activity as an almost-daily habit

- Practice developing a Colorado Mind-Set and tweaking your physical and social environments

WHAT TO EAT

As we explained in Chapter 5, the foods you eat during phase 1 are those that are low in energy density (to keep your hunger in check) and those that are not easily stored as fat. We call these Mile-High Metabolism foods, and you'll find a list of them on page 120. We show you step-by-step how to create satisfying, flavorful meals by mixing and matching the foods on this list. This way of eating may feel foreign to you at first, but if you go with it, you will reap the weight-loss rewards (and remember, it's only 2 short weeks!).

Even though your food selections are fairly limited during this phase, there's no need to subsist on ho-hum broiled chicken breast and a side of plain steamed broccoli. You can use unlimited amounts of herbs and spices (fresh or dried), aromatics (like onions, garlic, and shallots), vinegars, and lemon and lime juice to tantalize your taste buds. (You'll find cooking tips and recipes for all phases of the

Colorado Diet in Chapter 10.) And because the diet contains plenty of low-energy-density foods, most people don't feel hungry, especially after the initial 24 to 48 hours. Many of our patients have even reported feeling more energized on this diet.

Here are the rules for phase 1:

1.   **EAT SIX TIMES A DAY.** Space your meals and snacks so you're eating every 2 to 4 hours.

2.   **HAVE BREAKFAST WITHIN AN HOUR OF WAKING UP.**

3.   **DON'T COUNT CALORIES, MEASURE PORTIONS.** Make sure you have measuring cups and spoons at the ready. A digital scale can also be helpful.

4.   **HAVE THE RIGHT CARB AND PROTEIN MIX AT EVERY MEAL.** Pick one option from the Reignite Carbohydrates list and one from the Leanest Proteins list. Remember, you should choose a vegetable carbohydrate as your only carb for three of your meals.

5.   **EAT A HEALTHY FAT TWICE A DAY.**

The Leanest Proteins

— Beef

Serving size: 4–6 ounces

Not all red meat is created equal. In this phase, you eat only the leanest cuts of beef—those with fewer than 6 grams of fat in 4 ounces. These meats include top sirloin, flank, and extra-lean ground beef.

— Chicken and Turkey Breast
Serving size: 4–6 ounces

Boneless, skinless chicken and turkey breast are among the leanest sources of protein, and they are very versatile. You can bake, grill, or roast them. You can also buy lean ground turkey or chicken breast, as long as it is only breast meat with no skin or other parts included. Look for the words *lean ground turkey breast* or *lean ground chicken breast* on the package, then check the food label to make sure it contains no more than 4 grams of fat in 4 ounces.

— Fish
Serving size: 4–6 ounces

We recommend having very lean fish in this phase—tuna, cod, halibut, snapper, mahi mahi, haddock, and tilapia. The exception is salmon. Even though it's higher in fat than the other fish, its fats are the healthy kind. Still, count salmon as both a lean protein source *and* one of your fat servings for that day. As always, measure the portion size of your fish—especially with the salmon, since it's higher in calories, and a small portion error could add up to a big calorie difference. Bake, broil, or grill, but don't use any butter or sauce (fish is so flavorful, you don't need it anyway). Several of the recipes in Chapter 10 give you examples of other ways to flavor your fish.

— Egg Whites
Serving size: I cup (5–6 whites)

Egg whites should become a staple for your new lifestyle. They contain only lean protein, without any fat, and are easy to use in a number of ways. Elite athletes, who are always seeking good protein sources, routinely incorporate egg whites into their diets. You can either crack a whole egg and remove the yolk or purchase pasteurized egg whites in the carton. They're easy to cook—simply microwave them in a bowl or a mug—and they're versatile. You can change the flavor easily by adding salsa, hot sauce, and different veggies. See Chapter 10 for suggestions.

— Nonfat Plain Greek Yogurt
Serving size: 8 ounces

Nonfat Greek yogurt has almost twice the protein (15 to 20 grams in 6 ounces) of regular nonfat yogurt (9 grams in 6 ounces), making it an optimum lean protein source for phase 1. Note that we're recommending *plain nonfat* Greek yogurt. Flavored Greek yogurts are packed with added sugar, whereas plain Greek yogurt contains only the sugar that's naturally present in the milk, about 8 grams per 6 ounces versus 16 to 20 grams in fruit- or honey-flavored varieties. Phase 1 eliminates added sugar and minimizes natural sugar for a very good reason: Sugar inhibits fat-burning. Once you fix your metabolism, you can opt for fruit yogurt again or, better yet, add some fresh fruit to your plain yogurt, but for now stick with nonfat plain Greek yogurt. Before you freak out (yes, we've seen many of our patients make a yucky face when we recommend plain yogurt), know that you can temper the sour flavor of plain yogurt pretty easily. For a sweet hit, try flavoring it with fruit-flavored Crystal Light, MiO liquid water enhancer, 1 tablespoon of a sugar-free jelly, or any no-calorie sweetener. If you are lactose intolerant or otherwise sensitive to dairy, skip the yogurt and select a different protein from the list.

(continued on page 108)

HOLLY'S TIPS

Boosting Flavor

It's important to enjoy what you're eating. Although you are on phase 1 for just a short time, these foods form the foundation of the Colorado Diet, and they will be part of your eating plan for life. That's why I encourage you to stock up on herbs, spices, extracts, vinegars, artificial sweeteners, and certain condiments. Most of the items on the list below can be eaten freely because they have no calories. For certain items, I specify portions—because even low-calorie foods can stall weight loss if you overconsume them.

- Most dry seasonings, such as sea salt, black pepper, garlic salt, cinnamon, cumin, chili pepper, lemon pepper
- Lemon juice or lime juice (2 tablespoons per meal)
- Fresh garlic
- Flavor extracts: vanilla, mint, almond, lemon, root beer, butter, coconut, etc.
- Condiments: 2 tablespoons spicy mustard, reduced-sugar ketchup, sriracha sauce, hot sauce, nonfat mayonnaise; 1 tablespoon reduced-fat mayonnaise
- Nonstick cooking spray
- Sugar-free flavorings (for example, Crystal Light, MiO liquid water enhancers, Dasani Drops, Capella Flavor Drops)
- Sugar-free syrups (for example, DaVinci Gourmet sugar-free syrups, Torani sugar-free syrups)
- Most balsamic vinegars (1 tablespoon and under 40 calories)

- Sugar-free jams or jellies (1 tablespoon and 15 calories)
- PB2 natural defatted powdered peanut butter (2 tablespoons and 45 calories)
- Fat-free, sugar-free gelatin desserts
- Instant reduced-calorie puddings used as a flavoring only (1 tablespoon in a smoothie or recipe)
- Low-calorie sweeteners, like aspartame, stevia, and sucralose

Some people worry about the safety of low-calorie sweeteners, but they have been through more scientific testing than most foods in our diets, and they are approved by the FDA. Both the American Heart Association and the American Diabetes Association have published statements supporting the judicious use of these sweeteners as a tool to decrease sugar consumption in weight-reducing diets. Even more important, National Weight Control Registry members are consistent users of noncaloric sweeteners.

It's up to you whether or not to use these sweeteners. If you don't feel comfortable using them, don't. We believe they are safe, and they don't promote weight gain like sugars do. If you need more sweetness to help you savor your food, go ahead and try them—but in moderation. If you lace all your food with intense sweetness, you'll never get the chance to enjoy the wonderful range of flavors that exist in nature.

— Fat-Free Cottage Cheese
Serving size: 8 ounces

Like Greek yogurt, fat-free cottage cheese is a lean, easy source of protein that doesn't require cooking, so it gives you more flexibility. Look for cottage cheese that has less than 1 gram of fat, zero added sugar or fruit, and no more than 12 grams of natural sugar per 8 ounces.

— Protein Powder
Serving size: 1 scoop

Finding a lean protein source for six meals or snacks each day can be challenging. There are some meals, such as breakfast (think breakfast cereal, muffins, or smoothies), that don't contain sufficient protein unless you eat them with a concentrated source like meat or fish. In such cases, you can arrive at the protein level we believe is best for metabolism by adding protein powder. It's convenient, since it requires no cooking, refrigeration, or prep time. It's perfect when you travel. Use it to make shakes and smoothies, or add it to a variety of dishes.

Look for a protein powder that's made from a whey or a casein blend with 20 to 30 grams of protein per scoop. Avoid those brands that contain "bonus" ingredients, extra vitamins or minerals, or additives promising amazing muscle growth or fat loss. Also skip those with carbohydrates or fats mixed in. You just want pure protein. Added flavor is fine, as long as it doesn't contain added sugar (noncalorie sweeteners are okay). Common flavors include chocolate and vanilla, and some brands even come in flavors like cinnamon roll or raspberry truffle. These can be a nice treat when making a protein pancake or a dessert-style protein smoothie. Most regular grocery stores offer several brands, so you don't need to go to a supplement or health food store to find one.

Reignite Carbohydrates

— Oatmeal
Serving size: ½ cup dry old fashioned oats; ¼ cup dry steel cut oats (uncooked)

Choose these varieties over instant or quick-cooking oatmeal. Avoid any products with added sugar. If you like your oatmeal sweet, add a scoop of flavored protein powder and a noncalorie sweetener to the cooked oats. For a protein hit with a creamy texture, mix in some fat-free cottage cheese.

HOLLY'S TIPS

My Favorite Food Tricks: Greek Yogurt Cream Cheese

Like pumpkin, Greek yogurt cream cheese can trick your taste buds into thinking you're eating something rich and luscious, but it's actually very low in fat. Yogurt cheese is a terrific substitute for many high-fat items, such as sour cream, cream cheese, and even frosting! It's very easy to make; we give you the simple recipe on page 221. I like to think of it as a cheat food that isn't!

— Fat-Free Milk or Almond Milk
Serving size: 1 cup

Although fat-free milk and almond milk provide a combination of carbohydrate and protein, we are counting them as a carbohydrate source. Chocolate or vanilla flavors of almond milk are fine, as long as 1 cup has 35 to 45 calories and no added sugar. Almond milk typically has 3 to 4 grams of fat in 8 ounces and only a little protein and carbohydrate. Fat-free milk should have zero grams of fat and about 80 calories per cup. Mix either with a scoop of protein powder and

HOLLY'S TIPS *Try PB2, Powdered Peanut Butter*	My patients love PB2, and so do I. It's so popular that we began carrying it in our health and wellness center retail store here at the University of Colorado. It's got all the flavor of real peanut butter with 85 percent less fat and a fraction of the calories. I use it to flavor my protein smoothies, oatmeal, and protein pancakes. I even mix it into my Greek yogurt or cottage cheese. It comes in two flavors, regular and chocolate. If you are a peanut butter lover, this extra is a must-try for you. You can find it online or in some specialty stores. Visit the Bell Plantation Web site (bellplantation.com) and use the store locator to find a retailer that stocks PB2 in your area.

ice to make a smoothie with a satisfying, creamy texture, as we do in our Mile-High Protein Smoothie on page 208.

— Pumpkin
Serving size: 1 cup mashed

Pumpkin is the only starchy vegetable that's allowed in phase 1. It is high in fiber and, when used in recipes, imparts a texture that "fools" your taste buds: The dish will taste as if it's high in fat even though it isn't. Pumpkin also is a carbohydrate source that most people usually aren't tempted to overeat. Our patients love it. If you buy pumpkin in a can, make sure you're buying 100 percent pure pumpkin, not sweetened pumpkin pie mix. It should have about 80 calories per cup. Try it in pancakes, as a side dish, or even chili (see the recipes on pages 180 and 194).

— Vegetables
Serving size: No limit

Most vegetables—see the list on page 121—are high in nutrients and fiber and low in calories, which makes them perfect carbohydrate sources—as long as you don't fry them, drizzle them with butter, or drown them in oil or cheese. Eat them raw, steamed, baked, broiled, or roasted. If you don't want to bother with cutting and cleaning, look for veggies that come prewashed and precut in microwave steamer bags. Try different vegetables as you progress through the phases of the Colorado Diet. Your taste buds may adapt over time, so if there are types you didn't like in the first phases, consider giving them a second chance later.

Only the Healthiest Fats

— Almonds and Walnuts
  Serving size: 15–18 almonds or 8–9 walnut halves (Count them!)

During phase 1, you can have some almonds or walnuts as a fat serving. Look for 100-calorie snack packs—the portion is perfect every time.

HOLLY'S TIPS	When I start my morning with a bowl of cereal and fruit, I inevitably end up fighting hunger the
My Hunger-Busting Breakfast	rest of the day. But when I eat a protein-packed meal, I feel satisfied, and I'm not tempted to stray from my eating plan all day. One of my favorite options is a bowl of oatmeal and a side of five or six egg whites. I used to think this sounded bland, but now I love it. I flavor the egg whites in different ways—salsa, peppers, spinach, garlic powder, taco seasoning, Dijon mustard—depending on my mood. Sometimes I combine raw ground oats with the egg whites, add a little baking powder and vanilla extract, and cook them like a pancake. There are lots of variations of this type of recipe. Try the Cinnamon-Pumpkin Protein Pancakes on page 180.

— Olive Oil and Canola Oil
Serving size: 1 tablespoon

A drizzle on the bottom of your pan is always more than you think, so be sure to measure first. Try mixing 1 tablespoon of olive oil and 2 tablespoons of flavored or plain balsamic vinegar to make a dressing to serve over vegetables or salad. Save the oil for when you really need it for flavor or texture. If you need to use oil in cooking, use a little nonstick spray, which does not count toward your daily fat servings.

FREQUENTLY ASKED PHASE 1 QUESTIONS

What if I get hungry?

If you want a specific food (probably something sweet or salty), chances are you're experiencing a craving, not genuine hunger. Go for a walk or call a friend and see if the craving passes. Better yet, focus on your mood and remind yourself that eating really won't make negative feelings go away. We're conditioned to head for the refrigerator or the nearest drive-thru whenever we sense a craving or an uncomfortable emotion (boredom, sadness, anger, frustration etc.). But what happens if you don't give in and eat? Interestingly, most of the time the "feeling" disappears in a few minutes.

You can train yourself to get in touch with your body's appetite mechanism. When you feel hungry outside of regular meal times, sit with it for 15 to 20 minutes. "Real" hunger will get stronger during this period. If it's not hunger, the sensation will diminish and disappear. Not hitting the fridge or cupboards at the first twinge of hunger signals the body to dig into its fat stores to refuel itself. This is what happens when you're sleeping or when you let the hunger pangs pass.

If you're truly hungry, you'll be willing to satisfy your appetite with any one of a number of healthy foods. (A craving, in contrast, means you want a particular taste of food.) Try eating a 4-ounce serving of lean protein. Protein is the most satiating energy source, and a small protein-rich snack like chicken breast or Greek yogurt should tame your hunger until your next meal.

What should I drink?

Avoid any beverage with calories, unless it's a protein smoothie (made with phase 1 ingredients) counted as a meal or snack, or a glass of unsweetened almond or fat-free milk counted as a carbohydrate. No juice, sodas, or sports drinks. Calorie-free drinks like coffee or tea (you can add a splash of fat-free milk and/or artificial sweetener if you'd like, but no cream or sugar), sparkling or still water, diet sodas, or zero-calorie flavored waters are all fine. We recommend drinking 2 cups of water before each meal and a total of 10 cups a day to help control appetite.

Alcoholic beverages, when consumed in moderation, can add enjoyment to your diet and may confer health benefits, including a reduced risk of heart disease, stroke, and gallstones. But alcohol also has a lot of calories. In fact, a recent report from the Centers for Disease Control and Prevention found that Americans get as many calories from alcohol as from soft drinks. Alcohol has 7 calories per gram, so it is much closer in caloric density to fat (9 calories per gram) than to carbohydrate (4 calories per gram). One ounce or a shot of

80 proof whiskey, one 12-ounce beer, and one 5-ounce glass of wine each contain about 17 grams of alcohol, which would contribute 119 calories to your daily intake. For these reasons, we don't include alcohol in phase 1. After you've fixed your metabolism, you can add some alcohol back into your diet. Make it part of your indulgence meals in phases 2 and 3.

HOW TO MOVE

Moving your body will begin the process of unclogging your drain and help your metabolism become more flexible and better able to adjust to different types of foods. Your activity plan in phase 1 is easy—just start moving! Our research suggests that there's a basic threshold of activity (70 minutes per day) that's necessary to rebuild your metabolism, but you have multiple ways to accomplish this, and you don't have to reach that target overnight.

In these first 2 weeks, we simply want you to get in the habit of planning activity and become comfortable moving. Your goal is to make movement a basic part of your day, like brushing your teeth, watching the news, reading the paper, or calling your mom or sister on the phone.

In week 1, your goal is to plan a 10-minute session of activity for 6 days a week. It can be walking or anything that gets you moving. In week 2, you increase that to 15 minutes per day. That's it. If you want to do a bit more than 10 or 15 minutes, you can—but don't overdo it. If you are already regularly active, continue with your current amount of exercise.

It doesn't matter when you do your 10 to 15 minutes of activity. The important thing is that you find a place for it in your daily routine. In phase 2, you'll slowly increase your activity to the amount needed to rebuild your metabolism, and you'll pick one of two activity plans to fit your lifestyle. In this phase, however, the emphasis is simply on making room for movement in your life.

THINK THIN

Now that you know what to eat and how to move, it's time to work on developing the Colorado Mind-Set we discussed in Chapter 3. Remember that if you have a Colorado Mind-Set, it will be easier to stick with your lifestyle changes—in both the short and long term. Here in phase 1, we identify six simple exercises that can jump-start your efforts to develop the right frame of mind and a supportive environment.

Make sure you continue to work on finding your internal motivation as well as strengthening your willpower muscle. We build on these concepts in the future phases. Don't skip these activities! While you can lose weight short term without doing them (the diet is doing the heavy lifting in the Reignite phase), they become more and more important as you move toward where you need to be to maintain a healthy weight for years to come.

1. **Reconnect with your purpose and establish and post your whys.** The connection between your life purpose and your weight loss can provide an unwavering

source of motivation. Go back to the whys you wrote down when you were reading Chapter 3 and make a list of them to post in various places or carry with you. Tape your list of motivations to your refrigerator, desk, bathroom mirror, and clothes closet. Make a copy to carry with you in your wallet or purse. This makes your goals real and meaningful and serves as a constant reminder of your important reasons for adopting the Colorado Diet and lifestyle.

2. **Focus on the positive.** Imagine how you will feel when you lose your first 10 pounds. We see greater success in our patients who are able to emphasize the benefits of losing weight (such as feeling better and getting compliments from friends) rather than zero in on the negatives (feeling hungry or having sore muscles). The more you practice being positive, the easier it will become.

3. **Boost your willpower.** As we explained in Chapter 3, habits, routines, and rituals strengthen and preserve your willpower. Now develop one of these to help you stick with your diet and another to make daily physical activity easier to achieve. Consider the barriers preventing you from accomplishing the eating and activity behaviors outlined in this phase. What routines or rituals will help you overcome these barriers? Think about what will work for *you,* not your best friend or neighbor. The more specific you can be, the better. Will eating breakfast be a problem because you don't have time to make food in the morning *and* get your kids off to school? If so, set a routine to prepare a

healthy breakfast the night before so it's ready and waiting when you wake up. Or get in the habit of setting your alarm 10 minutes earlier so you have additional time to eat. Will preparing three meals with veggies as your Reignite carbohydrate source be an issue because doing the washing and chopping at the end of a long workday seems impossible? Make prepping veggies for the week ahead a Sunday routine or, better yet, make it a ritual and tie it to something that has additional meaning or purpose for you. For example, put on your favorite music or enlist your spouse, child, or best friend to assist you and use the time to catch up. Will you skip workouts in the evening because it's cold and dark when you get home? Then get into the routine of being active in the morning or find an indoor place to walk that's on the way home. Your routines and rituals will save your mental energy and keep your willpower muscle strong.

If you're having trouble thinking of options, consult Appendix II on page 253 for ideas and inspiration. But remember, the best habits, routines, and rituals are specific to you and your situation. Think about it, be creative, ask others, and have fun. You can do this.

4. **Do a kitchen audit.** Start by cataloging the foods you keep on hand all the time, both staples and snacks. Next, compare your list with the list of phase 1 foods and see how many of these Colorado Diet–friendly foods you stock routinely and which ones you will need to buy. Look at your spices and "extras": What

do you have on hand, and what might you pick up to add flavor to your dishes? You might buy three new spices and identify a new veggie recipe to try each week. We direct you to a tool for your kitchen audit in Resources on page 227. Make a phase 1 list of things you need.

After doing the audit, take action to change your food environment to support your new healthy eating plan. It's much easier to resist munching on a bag of chips if there are no chips in your cupboard, so this means throwing out the junk, the sugar, and the high-fat items. And it will likely mean a trip to the store to stock up on your new staples.

5. **Look at the people in your life.** Just as you did with the kitchen audit, take an inventory of the people in your life who will be supportive of your new lifestyle—family, friends, neighbors, coworkers. Tell the people who are supportive what your goals are and strive to use them as your social support system during the next 2 weeks.

6. **Start a food and exercise journal.** Keeping track of what you eat and when and what you did for exercise serves several purposes. It keeps you accountable, it helps you plan your healthy meals, and it allows you to refer to what worked best as you progress. It also provides a black-and-white record of all you've accomplished—and that's a powerful motivator. Write this information down in a notebook or type it into your laptop, smartphone, or tablet—whichever is more convenient.

Phase I Mile-High Metabolism Foods
Weeks 1–2

If a food isn't on this list, don't eat it—period—during the 2 weeks of phase I.

THE LEANEST PROTEINS
Have one at every meal and snack.

MEAT & POULTRY

Beef, ground, extra-lean (4–6 oz)

Beef, lean cuts (4–6 oz)

Chicken breast, without skin (4–6 oz)

Turkey breast, without skin (4–6 oz)

Turkey breast, lean ground (4–6 oz)

FISH

Cod (4–6 oz)

Mahi mahi (4–6 oz)

Salmon* (4–6 oz)

Snapper (4–6 oz)

Tilapia (4–6 oz)

Tuna (4–6 oz)

White fish (4–6 oz)

Salmon also counts as one fat.

EGG & HIGH-PROTEIN DAIRY

Cottage cheese, fat-free (8 oz)

Egg whites (1 cup or 5–6 whites)

Greek yogurt, nonfat plain (8 oz)

OTHER

Protein powder (1 scoop)

REIGNITE CARBOHYDRATES
Have one at a maximum of three meals and snacks.

GRAINS

Oats, steel-cut (¼ cup dry) or
old-fashioned rolled (½ cup dry)

DAIRY & DAIRY SUBSTITUTES

Almond milk, unsweetened (1 cup)   Fat-free milk (1 cup)

STARCHY VEGETABLES

Pumpkin (1 cup mashed)

VEGETABLE CARBOHYDRATES

These should be your only carb source at three meals or snacks a day.
However, you can have as much and as many of them as you like. You can
also have them in addition to Reignite Carbs at any meal.

Artichoke	Eggplant
Asparagus	Fennel
Beets	Green beans
Broccoli	Mushrooms
Brussels sprouts	Onions, scallions
Cabbage and Chinese cabbage (such as bok choy)	Parsnips
Carrots	Peppers, sweet and hot
Cauliflower	Salad greens—all varieties
Celery	Summer squash
Cucumbers	Tomato and tomato sauce
Dark leafy greens (collards, kale, spinach, Swiss chard)	Turnips and rutabagas
	Zucchini

ONLY THE HEALTHIEST FATS

Include fat in two meals or snacks per day.

NUTS

Almonds (15–18)   Walnuts (8–9 halves)

OILS

Canola oil (1 Tbsp)   Olive oil (1 Tbsp)

Rebuild Your Metabolism:
The Colorado Diet Phase 2 (Weeks 3–8)

CHAPTER 7

YOU'VE REIGNITED YOUR FAT burners. You've lost a good deal of weight, have more energy, and want to keep your momentum going. You're ready for phase 2. In these 6 weeks, you'll train your metabolism to use even more energy, further increase its capacity to burn fat, and develop the ability to switch rapidly between fuel sources. At the end of this phase, your metabolism will be primed to adjust to fluctuations in your diet (the condition known as metabolic flexibility). While phase 1 opened your clogged drain, phase 2 keeps it open and makes the drain bigger permanently!

Phase 2 lasts 6 weeks because in our experience, that's how long it takes to strengthen your metabolism if you've been relatively sedentary. You'll gradually increase your daily physical activity to

70 minutes per day, 6 days per week. At the same time, you'll continue eating from a list of select foods, but you'll have more choices than you did in phase 1. This is a fun phase, where you'll find out just how good it feels to move your body regularly and discover what happens when your old, stuck metabolism operates the way it was meant to. And you'll continue to melt off excess fat—typically, people lose 8 to 12 pounds in phase 2. You'll also become more aware of how your attitude and environment influence your weight and health, and you'll take further steps to support your Colorado Mind-Set so your lifestyle changes become easier and permanent.

PHASE 2 GOALS

- Continue losing weight by eating only the foods we recommend for phase 2

- Rebuild your metabolism by slowly increasing your activity level to 70 minutes a day

- Continue to develop your Colorado Mind-Set and physical and social environment to bolster your new lifestyle

WHAT TO EAT

The phase 2 food plan slowly and methodically adds more healthy foods without stopping your fat-burning weight loss. You can eat all the foods you enjoyed in phase 1, plus certain whole grains and fruits along with additional lean proteins and healthy fats. You'll burn all the calories you consume, along with more of your stored body fat.

The biggest change you'll notice in phase 2 is in your expanded carbohydrate choices; we call these Rebuild carbs. Because you're now using more calories and your appetite is aligning with your metabolism, we're less concerned that these carbs will prompt over-eating and fat storage. Think of your metabolism as a small fire. You can place small pieces of wood on the fire, one at a time, to stoke it and keep it going—but if you were to insert a large log from the get-go, you'd smother the tiny flames. So that we don't smother your fat-burning, we want you to incorporate these new carbs at only two of your six meals.

You can add Rebuild carbs in any order you like. If your weight loss stops when you eat a new food, that means your body may not be quite ready for that food. Turn to a different Rebuild carbohydrate; you can try the first one again in a few weeks as your metabolism strengthens.

As in phase 1, a vegetable carbohydrate must be your carb choice for three of your six meals. In phase 2, you're now allowed one planned indulgence meal per week. (We'll explain this in a minute.)

Here are the phase 2 rules:

1.   **EAT SIX TIMES A DAY.** Space your meals so you are eating every 2 to 4 hours.

2.   **HAVE BREAKFAST WITHIN AN HOUR OF WAKING UP.**

3.   **DON'T COUNT CALORIES, MEASURE PORTIONS.** If you think you have a handle on the portion sizes of phase 1 foods, then you no longer have to measure them. Do measure the new foods you add in this phase. If weight loss stops, go back to measuring all your foods.

4. **HAVE THE RIGHT CARB AND PROTEIN MIX AT EVERY MEAL.**
Each of your six meals should contain one lean protein
and one carbohydrate. Your protein choices have
expanded, and you can pick from either the phase 1 or
phase 2 Leanest Proteins lists. For two of those meals,
choose a Rebuild carb; for the other four, stick with
Reignite carbs. Remember, nonstarchy vegetables
should be your only carb at three of your meals.

5. **EAT A HEALTHY FAT TWICE A DAY.** Pick any fat from either
the phase 1 or phase 2 Only the Healthiest Fats list.

The Leanest Proteins

We expand the selection of protein choices in phase 2, but the proteins are still very lean. Your metabolism isn't yet ready to handle the larger amounts of fat that come with other protein sources.

— Shellfish
Serving size: 4–6 ounces

Crab, shrimp, scallops, and lobster are allowed in this phase, but be sure to steam, boil, or grill them—no cooking with butter.

— Other Red Meats—Buffalo, Ostrich, and Venison
Serving size: 4–6 ounces

These types of red meat can be low in fat as long as you pick a lean cut—one that contains more than 5 grams of fat in 4 ounces.

— Pork

Serving size: 4–6 ounces of pork tenderloin; 4 ounces of Canadian bacon

Pork tenderloin, with 4 grams of fat in 4 ounces, is one of the leanest red meats.

— Whole Eggs

Serving size: 1 whole egg plus 3–4 egg whites

To get enough protein, you should combine a whole egg with egg whites. You should have no more than 1 whole egg per day, but you can have egg whites alone at another meal on the same day, if you'd like. Be sure to cook them without butter or oil.

Rebuild Carbohydrates

— Ezekiel Bread, Whole Grain Pita or Tortilla

Serving size: 1 slice Ezekiel bread; 1 pita or tortilla

For many of our clinic participants, weight loss slows once they begin eating bread again, so we don't want you to go back to regular bread just yet. But because many people miss bread, we've come up with a compromise: Ezekiel bread. This product is made from sprouted live grains, not flour. There is nothing magical about Ezekiel bread, and there is nothing bad about regular whole grain bread. It's just that in our experience, this unique, dense bread doesn't appear to interfere with weight loss in the metabolism-rebuilding phase. Maybe that's because the bread is usually sold

HOLLY'S TIPS

My Favorite Foods— Ezekiel Bread

I love bread. It's one food that's easy for me to overeat. To control my cravings, I switched to Ezekiel bread. I buy it frozen or pop a fresh loaf in the freezer as soon as I'm home from the grocery store. Freezing keeps the bread from going stale and makes me more conscious of the amount I'm eating. To me, this bread has a nutty taste with a touch of sweetness. I usually toast it and spread on a little sugar-free jam or PB2 or combine it with a lean protein for a satisfying and tasty meal.

By making it my routine to buy and keep only frozen Ezekiel bread in my house, I've found it much easier to stay with my plan.

frozen, so when you get it home, you put it in the freezer, and that limits spontaneous consumption. One slice should have 80 to 100 calories.

Whole grain tortillas and pitas are acceptable if you prefer them. Look for those with no more than 150 calories and at least 10 grams of fiber. Tortillas especially run the gamut in terms of calories, fat, and fiber, so you absolutely must read labels and choose carefully. You may have to look in several stores to find the perfect brand, but there are great ones out there.

— Barley

Serving size: ½ cup cooked

Barley is a versatile grain with a rich nutlike flavor and an appealing pasta-like consistency. Although it is most commonly used in soups, you can use it the same way you would rice, couscous, or any other grain.

— Brown Rice, Wild Rice, and Rice Cakes

Serving size: ½ cup cooked, or 2 rice cakes

Now you can start eating small amounts of brown or wild rice, but not white rice or regular sushi rice because they shut off fat burning quickly. We love rice cakes. They come in preportioned sizes, and most are made of brown rice. (Check the ingredient list closely). Flavored rice cakes are fine as long as they don't have more than 3 grams of added sugar per serving. Top a rice cake with some Greek yogurt cheese flavored with PB2 or vanilla and cinnamon for a tasty snack.

— Quinoa

Serving size: ½ cup cooked

Quinoa has more protein than any other grain—4 grams per ¼ cup cooked compared with 2½ grams in bulgur wheat and brown rice. However, quinoa is still predominantly carbohydrate, and that's the way we count it in this phase. Like some other Rebuild carbohydrates, it's easy to overeat, so measure it!

— Beans

Serving size: ½ cup regular beans or ⅓ cup fat-free refried beans

Beans, like quinoa, have some protein. But they're still primarily carbohydrate, and we count them this way. Calories per serving should be around 100 to 150.

— Sweet Potato and Winter Squash

Serving size: 4 ounces, or ½ cup mashed

These veggies are flavorful but also easy to overeat. Measuring portion size is crucial—just one sweet potato, for example, can weigh 10 ounces or more. Buying them frozen may be a good idea. Turn these veggies into something extra special by serving them mashed with cinnamon and grated orange peel, ginger and garlic, cumin and coriander, or sage. They are delicious cubed and roasted in the oven: The pieces caramelize, and the sweet flavors intensify.

— Fat-Free and Low-Fat Cheese

Serving sizes: 1–2 pieces reduced-fat string cheese (50 calories each), ½ cup part-skim ricotta cheese

Even though these low-fat cheeses have some protein, it isn't enough to count as a lean protein on our plan. Fat-free ricotta cheese does exist but can be difficult to find. Part-skim is acceptable.

HOLLY'S TIPS

Decoding Food Allergies

Many of my patients ask me about food allergies. They want to know if they could be allergic to wheat or dairy. Usually the answer is no. Although a few people are allergic to certain foods, I believe that most of the patients who ask about allergies are really looking for an answer to the question "Why is losing weight so hard for me?" I get it. I'm in this field because I wanted to know why I struggle with my weight. It's tempting to blame a single food group for your weight problem, but it's really not that simple. Food allergies are rarely the sole cause of obesity. However, I do believe some foods may hinder weight loss in certain individuals. Perhaps it's because that particular food promotes overeating, increases insulin, stimulates appetite, or even decreases energy. So I tell my patients that if a food doesn't work for them for any reason—it causes hunger, bloating, weight gain, headaches, whatever—stop eating it and see if the issues resolve. You don't need to see an allergist for specialized tests. Just eliminate that food and move on. If you can't eat wheat, then you can't eat wheat. That doesn't mean that other people can't enjoy the grain or that wheat is necessarily bad. It just means it isn't right for you.

— Select Fruits

Serving size: 1 medium apple; 1 medium grapefruit; 1 cup blueberries, strawberries, or raspberries

In phase 2, you can have a serving of one of these fruits at one meal per day—*always* in combination with a lean protein. Remember, you must include vegetables in a minimum of three meals a day, as your carbohydrate source. If you notice that you get hungry a few hours later on the days you eat fruit, or if your weight loss stalls, back off on fruit until your metabolism gets stronger.

Only the Healthiest Fats

In phase 2, we add a few more healthy fat options to increase variety and flavor in your diet. These fats are low in saturated fat and high in monounsaturated fat, which means they are the healthiest fats and tend to be burned for energy rather than stored as body fat. We still want to keep fat sources controlled in this phase, because even healthy fat has 9 calories in every gram (versus 4 calories per gram for protein and carbohydrate).

— Avocado

Serving size: 1/3 of a medium avocado

Avocados are very satisfying, thanks to their cool, creamy texture and fiber content. Usually recipes call for raw avocado, and the fruit can turn an unappetizing brown once it's peeled and exposed to air. Sprinkling it with a little lemon or lime juice helps it keep its bright green color.

— Olives
Serving size: 10 small or 5 medium/large olives

These ancient fruits are very versatile. There come in wide variety of types and flavors—from the ubiquitous canned black olives to the tiny purple niçoise to the big green Greek olives stuffed with pimiento—and they can be used as a condiment or appetizer, tossed in salads, or ground into spreads. Like olive oil, they are a good source of heart-healthy monounsaturated fats and antioxidants.

— Pistachios
Serving size: 25 pistachios

Pistachios in the shell are a great nut to snack on when you're trying to lose weight. The act of shelling them slows you down so you're aware of how many you're eating and you don't just gobble them up mindlessly. They also have fewer calories than other nuts.

A NEW RULE: HAVE A WEEKLY INDULGENCE MEAL

As your metabolism becomes more flexible, your diet can become more varied. Beginning in phase 2, you can have one indulgence meal (note: not an indulgence *day*) a week. Indulgence meals serve a specific purpose. They remind you that no food is off-limits forever and that any food you want is no more than 7 days away. What you choose is up to you, but there is one tiny catch: You must plan for it! Don't simply walk into a bakery and buy a chocolate chip cookie just because it smells good and then claim in retrospect that it was your indulgence meal. Set the date in advance—looking forward to a treat is half the pleasure. Also, planning for your indulgence allows you to focus on flavors that you truly appreciate and enjoy the most. This can put you back in touch with the joy of eating and help you develop a healthy relationship with food.

HOLLY'S TIPS

Indulgence Meals and Your Mind-Set

Many of my patients fear that once they lose weight, they will never be able to eat their favorite food again. When this sense of deprivation sets in, they tend to get caught up in the *life is not fair; I should be able to eat a slice of pizza* rationalization. That leads them to focus on all the things they can't have instead of all the things they can, and they inevitably fall off the wagon. The weekly indulgence meal is a way to counter this negative mind-set. If you find yourself craving a piece of pizza, chocolate ice cream, or a glass of cold beer, you can plan to enjoy that treat at your next indulgence meal. Many of my patients find that their craving passes before their indulgence meal arrives. But if it's still there on their planned day, they're free to enjoy that food. That's the beauty of the Colorado Diet— you never feel deprived.

HOW TO MOVE

By the completion of phase 2, you will be moving for 70 minutes per day, 6 days each week. You'll take 1 day off to rest and recover. If this sounds like a lot, don't worry: We'll get you to the 70-minute goal gradually. You'll see how easy it can be to make activity part of your day. You can also reread Chapter 4 to motivate yourself and establish a positive mind-set.

In Chapter 4, we introduced the two approaches to becoming more active: the Structured Plan and the Flexible Plan. The Structured Plan focuses on planned physical activity. The Flexible Plan allows you to combine measured lifestyle activity (like taking the stairs or walking across the parking lot) with shorter sessions of planned exercise. Unless they have an extremely active job that keeps them walking or running all the time, very few people can reach the necessary activity goal through lifestyle movement alone. Either plan will work. Pick the one that best fits your life.

// The Structured Plan

If you've chosen the Structured Plan, you'll gradually increase your planned activity to 70 minutes a day. In the first week of phase 2, you move for 20 minutes per day. Every week thereafter, you increase your dose of exercise by 10 minutes a day. By the end of phase 2 (week 8), you'll be active 70 minutes daily. Take a look at the list of planned activities on page 75 and you'll see that we're talking about moderate-intensity activity, not necessarily all-out exertion. It's also important to remember that you can break up the planned activity into two or three bouts each day—while exercise needs to be planned, it does not have to be done in one continuous session. For instance, you can combine a 25-minute after-lunch walk with a 45-minute water aerobics class after work. Similarly, you can walk on Wednesdays and take a class on Fridays. Regardless of which planned activity you choose or when you decide to do it, you must commit to getting your daily minutes in before you go to bed at night. Make it a challenge. Check off your success each day as you feel your metabolism build.

// *The* Flexible Plan

If you've chosen the Flexible Plan, you'll gradually increase your lifestyle activity to 7,000 steps per day and slowly bring your planned physical activity up to 35 minutes a day. This combination is equivalent to about 70 minutes per day of planned activity.

Here's how to start. Clip on a pedometer first thing in the morning and then make sure you accomplish the required number of steps before you go to bed. No guessing! Just as most of us can't accurately gauge food portions, we're usually not very good at estimating how much we move. Start with a goal of 4,000 steps a day. Depending on how active you are right now, you may find that you're already at that level, or close to it, and upping your steps won't require much effort. Remove the pedometer during your planned activity—no double-dipping! We want the pedometer readings to accurately reflect your lifestyle activity only.

As the weeks pass and the step goals increase, almost everyone will need to boost their usual lifestyle activity to reach those 7,000 steps per day. We suggest looking at your pedometer throughout the day and changing your behavior accordingly to ensure that you hit your goal by bedtime. Don't let bedtime roll

Daily Activity Plan
(6 days/week)

WEEK	STRUCTURED PLAN PLANNED ACTIVITY	FLEXIBLE PLAN STEPS	FLEXIBLE PLAN PLANNED ACTIVITY
3	20 minutes/day	4,000 steps/day	15 minutes/day
4	30 minutes/day	5,000 steps/day	15 minutes/day
5	40 minutes/day	5,000 steps/day	20 minutes/day
6	50 minutes/day	6,000 steps/day	25 minutes/day
7	60 minutes/day	6,000 steps/day	30 minutes/day
8	70 minutes/day	7,000 steps/day	35 minutes/day

around only to find you're 3,000 steps short of your goal!

If you happen to be one of the very few people who already take 7,000 steps a day, that's great. Use the pedometer to ensure that you continue to meet your goal. You might strive to go a little higher—to 9,000 or even 10,000. When it comes to physical activity, the more the better. Be sure to write your steps and activity minutes in your journal.

FREQUENTLY ASKED PHASE 2 QUESTIONS

Do I need to follow the schedule?

Phasing in activity allows your body to adjust gradually to more movement and enables you to find time to fit movement into your life permanently. You may already be exercising, but it's unlikely you're at the recommended levels 6 days per week. If you're currently doing more than our plan suggests, great! We certainly don't want you to reduce your movement.

Instead, start with where you are and increase gradually. For example, if you've chosen the Structured Plan and are currently doing 30 minutes every day, you can start there and increase by 10 minutes a day each week. If you're occasionally active, but not on a regular basis, you'll strive to get in activity 6 days per week.

Can I pack all my weekly activity into 2 or 3 days?

It may be tempting to go on a 4-hour hike on Saturday and a 3-hour bike ride on Sunday and declare yourself done with exercise for the week. We don't recommend this approach. You're better able to maintain metabolic flexibility if you use your muscles every day. Some of the negative metabolic changes we discussed in Chapter 2 occur after just 24 hours of sedentary behavior. A weekend hike is great, but even if it lasts 3 hours, count it as 1 day's worth of activity.

What if I miss a day?

There will be weeks when you simply can't fit in all your planned activity. That's okay, as long as those periods are the exception, not the norm. When you miss a session, don't beat yourself up—just get back on track the next day. It's especially important not to miss 2 days in a row. If you feel up to it, try to do a little more activity the next day to make up for the missed time. Don't use one day's failure as an excuse to give up. People in Colorado and participants in the National Weight Control Registry wake up each morning and think about how they will get their activity that day. If you make movement a routine and a ritual, you'll be like those folks, and you won't miss many days.

THINK THIN

In phase 2, you continue developing the Colorado Mind-Set and adjusting your environment so that your new, healthy behaviors are easier to maintain.

1. **NOTICE WHAT'S CHANGED.** As you lose weight and start to feel different, your mind-set and attitude will improve. How do these emotions alter the way you view your relationships, your job, and your recreation? How do they connect to your purpose? Use the positive energy you experience to build the confidence and determination to do the things that are most important in your life.

   One of our patients told us that her key reason for losing weight—her why—was to be able to reach down and tie her shoes. She didn't want to have to wear slip-on shoes or get someone to help her every time she needed to go outside. By the middle of phase 2 of the Colorado Diet, she had lost enough weight that tying her shoes was a breeze. She said she felt amazingly empowered and in control— a feeling she hadn't experienced in years. While her short-term goal (being able to tie her shoes unassisted) might seem simplistic and minor, it was actually her catalyst. She decided to volunteer at the community shelter and the children's hospital, something she had always wanted to do but had been embarrassed to attempt because of her limited mobility and low energy. The simple act of tying her shoelaces opened a door to many possibilities and to a life course she had been unable to visualize previously.

2. **DEVELOP A GRATITUDE ATTITUDE.** Take a few minutes every morning to write down something you are grateful for and looking forward to that day. No matter what your day has in store for you or what happened yesterday, there *is* something positive. You can be thankful for people, things, events, nature—anything, really. You may laugh at this, but on those brisk Colorado days, Holly is grateful that her car handles well in the snow and has awesome heated seats! Jim is often grateful for a friend, family member, or coworker. We both appreciate the beauty of the mountains we can see from our offices. You might be surprised by how pausing for just a few minutes every morning to note and enjoy what you have can take the sting out of some of your most difficult days. It really does help create a Colorado Mind-Set.

3. **ADD MORE ROUTINES AND RITUALS.** In phase 1, you created two routines or rituals, one for your diet and one for your physical activity. Keep practicing these and they will eventually become second nature. Over the next 6 weeks, we want you to add two more food and two more activity routines or rituals to your list. Turn to Appendix II on page 253 for ideas. By the end of phase 2, we'd like you to have a total of six routines or rituals in place, two from phase 1 and four you developed during phase 2. Write them down in your journal and practice them until they become your norm.

4. **DO AN EXERCISE AUDIT.** In phase 1, we asked you to audit your food environment. Now we want you to audit your physical activity environment. Start with your home and then look at

your neighborhood, community, and workplace. Do you have exercise equipment at home? Are there stairs in your house or apartment complex? Do you own a pedometer or an activity-monitoring device? Do you own a bike? Do you own a good pair of walking shoes? Do you have appropriate clothes for your activity? Do you own a dog? Is your neighborhood walkable? Is it safe? Are there parks or walking and bike paths? Is there a fitness club or recreation center nearby? A school with a track? A pool? Tennis courts? Are there places (such as malls) where you can walk indoors during rain or snow? What about your workplace? Does it have a workout room? Does your employer contribute toward a fitness club membership? Are there usable stairs? Places to walk nearby?

Use your audit to identify barriers and come up with an action plan for overcoming them. Look for ways you can change your environment to get more physical activity. Start with the easiest things first, like making sure you have good walking shoes and clothes. Buy a pedometer if you don't have one. We find that just wearing a pedometer tends to increase physical movement. Make some maps of your neighborhood to lay out good walking routes. Using your pedometer, determine how many steps each route takes and develop a "step map" of your surroundings. Map several routes of different lengths so you have multiple "step recipes" on hand to choose from to get to your daily total activity level if you're on the Flexible Plan. Once you have transformed your home environment, look for ways to move more in your workplace. When you start paying attention, you're likely to find ample opportunities to build extra action into your day.

By the way, this audit will strengthen your willpower muscle: The planning and documenting help take all those willpower-draining decisions out of the equation.

5.   **MAKE A HEALTHY DATE.** Dust off that list of people in your life whom you identified as sources of support in phase 1. Now think of ways of socializing with these folks that mesh with your new lifestyle. Perhaps sharing a healthy meal or a walk in the park? How about a bike ride on the weekend or a day at the zoo walking to all the exhibits? Enlisting them in planning a healthy progressive dinner? There are many ways you can incorporate health into your social life.

Phase 2 Mile-High Metabolism Foods
Weeks 3–8

During these 6 weeks, you can choose foods from this list. **Boldface** references foods added in this phase.

THE LEANEST PROTEINS
Have one at every meal and snack.

MEAT & POULTRY

Beef, ground, extra-lean (4–6 oz)	**Ostrich, lean cuts (4–6 oz)**
Beef, lean cuts (4–6 oz)	**Pork tenderloin (4–6 oz)**
Buffalo, lean cuts (4–6 oz)	Turkey breast, without skin (4–6 oz)
Canadian bacon (4 oz)	Turkey breast, lean ground (4–6 oz)
Chicken breast, without skin (4–6 oz)	**Venison, lean cuts (4–6 oz)**

FISH

Cod (4–6 oz)	Mahi mahi (4–6 oz)
Crab (4–6 oz)	Salmon* (4–6 oz)
Lobster (4–6 oz)	**Scallops (4–6 oz)**

*Salmon also counts as one fat.

FISH—*CONTINUED*

Shrimp (4–6 oz)
Snapper (4–6 oz)
Tilapia (4–6 oz)

Tuna (4–6 oz)
White fish (4–6 oz)

EGG & HIGH-PROTEIN DAIRY

Cottage cheese, fat-free (8 oz)
Eggs, whole (1, plus 3–4 egg whites)

Egg whites (1 cup or 5–6 whites)
Greek yogurt, nonfat plain (8 oz)

OTHER

Protein powder (1 scoop)

REBUILD CARBOHYDRATES
Have one at a maximum of three meals and snacks.

FRUIT

Apple (1 medium)
Berries (1 cup)

Grapefruit (1 medium)

BREADS

Ezekiel bread (1 slice)

Whole grain pita or tortilla (1)

GRAINS

Barley (½ cup cooked)
Brown or wild rice (½ cup cooked)
Rice cakes (2)

Oats, steel-cut (¼ cup dry) or old-fashioned rolled oats (½ cup dry)
Quinoa (½ cup cooked)

DAIRY & DAIRY SUBSTITUTES

Almond milk, unsweetened (1 cup)
Fat-free milk (1 cup)

Reduced-fat string cheese (1–2 pieces)
Fat-free or part-skim ricotta cheese (½ cup)

BEANS & STARCHY VEGETABLES

Beans (½ cup whole; ⅓ cup fat-free refried)
Pumpkin (1 cup mashed)

Sweet potato (4 oz, ½ cup mashed)
Winter squash (4 oz, ½ cup mashed)

(continued)

Phase 2 Mile-High Metabolism Foods—*Continued*

VEGETABLE CARBOHYDRATES

These should be your only carb source at three meals or snacks a day. However, you can have as much and as many of them as you like. You can also have them in addition to Rebuild Carbs at any meal.

Artichoke

Asparagus

Beets

Broccoli

Brussels sprouts

Cabbage and Chinese cabbage (such as bok choy)

Carrots

Cauliflower

Celery

Cucumbers

Dark leafy greens (collards, kale, spinach, Swiss chard)

Eggplant

Fennel

Green beans

Mushrooms

Onions, scallions

Parsnips

Peppers, sweet and hot

Salad greens—all varieties

Summer squash

Tomato and tomato sauce

Turnips and rutabagas

Zucchini

ONLY THE HEALTHIEST FATS

Include fat in two meals or snacks per day.

NUTS

Almonds (15–18)

Pistachios (25)

Walnuts (8–9 halves)

OILS

Canola oil (1 Tbsp)

Olive oil (1 Tbsp)

OTHER

Avocado (⅓ medium)

Olives (10 small or 5 medium/ large)

Reinforce Your Metabolism:
The Colorado Diet Phase 3 (Weeks 9–16)

CHAPTER 8

BY NOW, YOU'RE HALFWAY through the Colorado Diet. In the remaining 8 weeks, you'll continue to follow our specific diet and physical activity plans while you practice the skills needed to keep your weight off forever. You'll lose more weight *and* enjoy the benefits of your rebuilt metabolism. By the time they finish this phase, many of our patients say they feel like a new person—they have reinvented themselves—and that feeling is a powerful motivator. The increased metabolic flexibility you've achieved allows you to greatly expand the variety of foods you can eat. Remember how we said way back in Chapter 2 that when you have a Mile-High Metabolism, you can eat more food, not less? Here's where we prove it!

PHASE 3 GOALS

- Continue losing weight by eating only the foods we recommend

- Reinforce your new metabolism and keep it flexible by continuing to exercise 70 minutes per day

- Continue to develop your Colorado Mind-Set and physical and social environment

WHAT TO EAT

Phase 3 is all about solidifying your diet and increasing the number of good fuel foods you can eat. We still want you to limit foods that can slow weight loss—such as high-fat items like chips and high-sugar items like candy and sweets—but now you can continue to broaden the types of carbohydrates (breads, pasta, potatoes, corn, beans, fruits) in your diet. These carbohydrates would have shut off fat-burning when your metabolism was broken, but you can handle them now. And you'll get to enjoy *two* weekly indulgence meals.

You still need to watch portion sizes if you want to keep losing weight, but you'll have more leeway. Stick with your activity and movement goals and you'll be surprised at how much food you can enjoy. In fact, we *want* you to eat as much food as you can.

Here are the phase 3 rules:

1. **EAT SIX TIMES A DAY.** Space your meals so you are eating every 2 to 4 hours.

2. **HAVE BREAKFAST WITHIN AN HOUR OF WAKING UP.**

3. **DON'T COUNT CALORIES, MEASURE PORTIONS.** If you think you have a handle on the portion sizes of phase 1 and 2 foods, then you no longer have to measure them. Do measure the new foods you add in this phase. If you hit a weight-loss plateau, go back to measuring all your food.

4. **HAVE THE RIGHT CARB AND PROTEIN MIX AT EVERY MEAL.** Each of your six meals should contain one lean protein and one carbohydrate. Your protein choices have expanded, and you can pick from all three Leanest Protein lists. For three meals, your carbohydrate choice can be fruit, beans, dairy, or grains from the Reignite, Rebuild, or Reinforce carbohydrate lists. For the other three, you should still choose nonstarchy veggies as your only carbohydrate source. As in phase 2, pay attention when you're adding in a new carbohydrate source and monitor your hunger level and weight. If you notice an increase in cravings or appetite when you eat a certain carbohydrate, it may be that you'll need to limit that carbohydrate to your indulgence meal.

5. **EAT A HEALTHY FAT TWICE A DAY.** Pick any fat from any of the Only the Healthiest Fats lists.

The Leanest Proteins

— Beef
   Serving size: 4–6 ounces

Continue to pick lean cuts as you did in phases 1 and 2, but you can add New York strip steak and filet mignon to your list. These two cuts are a little higher in fat, but your metabolism is now flexible enough to process the fat. It's still best to keep your red meat fat count under 12 grams per 4 ounces. Choose cuts that have the least amount of visible fat or marbling. Save the fattest cuts of red meat (such as rib eye and T-bone) for your indulgence meals, or wait until you've completed phase 3.

— Turkey Bacon, Turkey Sausage, Lean Ham, and Lean Deli Meat
  Serving sizes: ½–1 cup turkey sausage; 2 turkey sausage patties; 4 slices turkey bacon; or 4–6 ounces lean ham or lean deli meat

We add these foods in phase 3 because they increase variety in your diet, and if you eat them in moderation, they won't make you gain weight. Look for meats that are low in fat and calories. Always read the labels. Some turkey sausage can have a lot of fat, and fat content varies considerably among brands. As a rule, choose products that have fewer than 6 or 7 grams of fat per serving. We like Jimmy Dean turkey sausage. It has 4 grams of fat in ½ cup of crumbles or 7 grams in two patties, and it comes precooked in a refrigerated bag. Sprinkle it into egg whites or wrap it in a high-fiber tortilla quesadilla.

We also like Healthy Ones Honey Smoked Turkey sliced to order at the deli counter. It has 100 calories and 2 grams of fat in 4 ounces. Healthy Ones offers a lean roast beef, too. As always, read the labels and make your best choice.

— Trout and Sea Bass
  Serving size: 4–6 ounces

Although these fish may have a bit more fat than the white fish in phases 1 and 2, they fit into your phase 3 healthy diet with your new metabolism. Just skip the butter when cooking!

— Nonfat or Low-Fat Flavored Greek Yogurt
Serving size: 8 ounces

Take your pick of flavors—fruit, vanilla, honey, etc.—just make sure you stay with a low-fat or nonfat variety. They are still a good source of protein. (Non-Greek or regular low-fat yogurts, plain or flavored, are included under Reinforce carbohydrates in this phase, since they have less protein and more carbohydrate.) Pay attention to what happens after you eat one, though. Some people are more sensitive to sugar than others. If you notice you're hungry shortly after eating flavored Greek yogurt (or regular yogurt), or you suddenly crave sugary foods, switch back to nonfat plain Greek yogurt.

— Protein Bars
Serving size: 1 bar (250 calories max)

While we would not suggest eating these bars too often, they are lean protein sources and great, easy snacks, especially when you're traveling. Their convenience factor makes them acceptable in phase 3. Holly always carries an emergency bar in her purse or coat pocket in case she's caught up longer than expected and in need of a meal. She's especially fond of Quest Bars, which are sold online at questproteinbar.com.

We recommend bars with a minimum of 15 to 20 grams of protein and fewer than 5 grams of sugar. Look for a minimum of 5 grams of fiber, but the more the better. The total calorie count should not exceed 250 calories. Make sure your bar meets these nutrition standards and isn't just a glorified candy bar. If you want one of the latter, have it during an indulgence meal and make it count—choose one you really love.

Reinforce Carbohydrates

— Whole Grain Bread and English Muffins
Serving size: 1 slice regular bread, 2 slices reduced-calorie bread, or 1 English muffin

Bread lovers, rejoice! Phase 3 allows you to reintroduce bread into your meal plan. Select a product made from 100 percent whole grains. Look for the word *whole* in the ingredient list. A slice of regular bread should have 100 calories; reduced calorie bread 45 to 50 calories. English muffins should have no more than 150 calories. We suggest taking a pass on the bread basket in restaurants unless it's your indulgence meal. Most people overeat from the basket before their meal even arrives. Use bread as part of your meal and enjoy it, but skip it as an appetizer.

— Whole Grain Bagel Thins
Serving size: 1 bagel thin

Everyone seems to love bagels. There are entire franchise chains across the country devoted to them. We love bagels, too. Unfortunately, most bagels are huge and not that healthy. Even the whole grain ones have a lot of calories—and it's hard to stop at half a bagel. With this in mind, we have found that whole grain bagel thins solve the portion problem. We like Thomas' 100% Whole Wheat Bagel Thin Bagels (110 calories). There are other brands on the market, and even one of the big bagel chains (Einstein Bros.) now offers thins. These slender versions of their bulky cousins are awesome for making breakfast sandwiches, mini pizzas, even buns for hamburgers. We recommend eating them with flavored yogurt cheese or with some melted low-fat cheese and turkey sausage or turkey bacon.

— Whole Grain Pasta
Serving size: ½–1 cup cooked

Pasta can spell trouble for many people. It's just too easy to overeat, and it's hard to fill up on a reasonably sized portion. We've also noticed that some of our patients' weight loss stalls when they eat pasta. But with your new metabolism, you can definitely try it and see how you do. Remember: Whole grain has more fiber than regular pasta, but it doesn't have fewer calories. Always measure pasta! It's easy to underestimate how much is on the plate. You're aiming for 1 cup cooked, max. Here's a trick to get more satisfaction out of a single serving of pasta: add vegetables. They will increase the bulk of your meal, make you feel more full, and add extra flavor and nutrients to the dish, too. Mix 1 cup of pasta with 1 to 2 cups of your favorite cooked vegetables and some protein, like chicken.

— Whole Grain Couscous
Serving size: ½–1 cup cooked

Couscous has approximately 175 calories per cooked cup. Use it the way you would beans, brown rice, or whole grain pasta. Mix it with veggies to increase the serving size of your side dish or meal.

— Baked Potato
Serving size: 1 medium (6–8 ounces)

Potatoes are a good carbohydrate source for active people when prepared without fatty toppings and in appropriate portions. They offer fiber, potassium, and vitamin C, especially if you eat the skin. Potatoes are often served with high-calorie and high-fat toppings (like butter or margarine, sour cream, or gravy) that pile on the calories and unhealthy fats. Flavor yours with salsa or a little low-fat cheese and a drizzle of olive oil. If you like mashed potatoes, cook them in low-sodium chicken broth to substitute for cream or butter. Red and Yukon Gold potatoes are also tasty sliced into quarters, tossed in a little olive oil, and roasted until browned. And weigh the potatoes before you buy them! Many top 16 ounces—that's two servings. Look for one about the size of your fist.

— Corn, Peas, and Edamame
Serving size: 1 cup or 1 medium ear corn, 1 cup peas, ½ cup shelled edamame

Now that your metabolism is working well, it more efficiently processes starchy carbs like corn, peas, and edamame, so you can add these to your meals for variety. It's almost impossible to overeat non-starchy vegetables, but if you're not careful, these starchy veggies you're adding can be overeaten and thus stall weight loss. So stick to the portion sizes we recommend.

— Fruit
Serving size: 1 piece, or 1 cup

In this phase, you can enjoy oranges, cherries, peaches, melons, bananas, apricots, mangos, kiwifruits, pears, and plums—actually, any fruit you like. When combined with some protein, fruit is especially useful before or after a big workout. Some people do fine with any kind of fruit once their activity level is high; others may need to limit certain types. As you add fruit, notice if you get hungry later in the day; if so, cut back. To begin, we recommend limiting fruit as your carbohydrate source to two meals per day. After a few weeks, if things are still good, you could increase that to three meals per day. Remember, vegetables should still be eaten with three of your daily meals. Veggies will always be your go-to carb source in any phase.

— High-Fiber, Low-Sugar Cereals
Serving size: 1 cup (150–200 calories)

Cold cereal is convenient and can be healthy, but it's easy to overeat. Pay attention to portion size. Look for cereals that have more than 8 grams of fiber per cup and are low in sugar (no more than 6 grams per cup). For example, Kashi GoLean has 10 grams of fiber per cup and only 6 grams of sugar. Another cereal that fits in well with the Colorado Diet is Fiber One Honey Clusters. One cup has 13 grams of fiber and 6 grams of sugar.

— Dairy

Serving size: 6–8 ounces nonfat or low-fat regular yogurt (plain or flavored), ¼ cup shredded or 1 ounce low-fat or reduced-fat cheese

Remember: Even though dairy has some protein, we count these foods as carbohydrates because they have far less protein than the selections in our Leanest Proteins category. Look for a regular yogurt that contains fewer than 200 calories and reduced-fat cheese that has 60 to 80 calories per serving and 6 grams of fat or fewer.

Only the Healthiest Fats

— Almond and Peanut Butters

Serving size: 1 tablespoon

These butters are packed with the same healthy monounsaturated fats as olive oil but taste much better than olive oil with low-sugar grape jelly! We did not include them in phase 1 because nut butters are frequently overeaten. You must measure these carefully; 1 tablespoon is not much. Remember, fat has 9 calories per gram, and protein and carbohydrate have just 4; therefore, anything that has a lot of fat is very calorie-dense: Even a small amount is packed with calories.

— Hummus

Serving size: ¼ cup

People often think of hummus as a source of protein because it contains chickpeas. However, it also contains olive oil and tahini, and therefore we consider it a fat. Use it sparingly, as you would a peanut butter or olive oil, and measure it. Like nuts and nut butters, hummus supplies good fats.

FREQUENTLY ASKED PHASE 3 QUESTIONS

What if my weight loss stalls?

First, know that if you meet your daily activity goal and stick to foods on the list, you'll start losing weight again. However, now that you've been on the Colorado Diet for a while, you may have become less attentive to portion sizes. Keep in mind that most successful weight-loss maintainers say their success is due in part to paying attention to what and how much they eat every day. To lose weight, some food restriction is required, but you won't have to keep restricting so much to keep the weight off.

Be especially aware of portion sizes of good fats (like almond or peanut butter) and grains (like brown rice and pasta). It's very easy to underestimate serving sizes of these foods. If your portion sizes seem correct, then look at the foods you most recently added to your diet. Try removing any that coincided with your plateau. It may require some trial and error, but this process of elimination will help identify any foods that your body doesn't metabolize well. If you're truly struggling, you can always fall back into phase 1 for a few days to restart your weight loss.

What if I totally fall off the wagon?

First, don't despair. Acknowledge that succeeding at weight loss takes effort, then give yourself a break. Don't use a few bad days—or even a few weeks—as an excuse to quit. Instead, focus on reaffirming your commitment to eating well and moving. If you need to, you can return to phase 1 for a few days or weeks until you've worked your way back.

Phase 3 Mile-High Metabolism Foods
Weeks 9–16

During these 8 weeks, you can choose foods from this list. **Boldface** references foods added in this phase.

THE LEANEST PROTEINS
Have one at every meal and snack.

MEAT & POULTRY

Beef, ground, extra-lean (4–6 oz)	**New York strip steak (4–6 oz)**
Beef, lean cuts (4–6 oz)	Ostrich, lean cuts (4–6 oz)
Buffalo, lean cuts (4–6 oz)	Pork tenderloin (4–6 oz)
Canadian bacon (4 oz)	**Turkey bacon (4 slices)**
Chicken breast, without skin (4–6 oz)	Turkey breast, without skin (4–6 oz)
Filet mignon (4–6 oz)	Turkey breast, lean ground (4–6 oz)
Lean deli meat (4–6 oz)	**Turkey sausage (½–1 cup or 2 patties)**
Lean ham (4–6 oz)	Venison, lean cuts (4–6 oz)

FISH

Cod (4–6 oz)	Shrimp (4–6 oz)
Crab (4–6 oz)	Snapper (4–6 oz)
Lobster (4–6 oz)	Tilapia (4–6 oz)
Mahi mahi (4–6 oz)	**Trout (6–8 oz)**
Salmon* (4–6 oz)	Tuna (4–6 oz)
Scallops (4–6 oz)	White fish (4–6 oz)
Sea bass (6–8 oz)	

*Salmon also counts as one fat.

EGG & HIGH-PROTEIN DAIRY

Cottage cheese, fat-free (8 oz)	Greek yogurt, nonfat plain (8 oz)
Egg whites (1 cup or 5–6 whites	**Greek yogurt, nonfat or low-fat, flavored (8 oz)**
Eggs, whole (1, plus 3–4 egg whites)	

OTHER

Protein bars (1 bar)	Protein powder (1 scoop)

REINFORCE CARBOHYDRATES
Have one at a maximum of three meals and snacks.

FRUIT

Apples (1 medium)

Apricots (3 fruit or 1 cup)

Banana (1 fruit or 1 cup)

Berries (1 cup)

Cherries (1 cup)

Dried cherries (1 ½ tablespoons)

Grapes (1 cup)

Grapefruit (1 medium)

Kiwifruit (1 fruit or 1 cup)

Mango (1 cup)

Orange (1 fruit or 1 cup)

Peach (1 fruit or 1 cup)

Pear (1 fruit or 1 cup)

Plum (1 fruit or 1 cup)

BREADS

Ezekiel bread (1 slice)

Rice cakes (2)

Whole grain bagel thins (1 bagel thin)

Whole grain bread (1 slice regular or 2 slices reduced-calorie) or English muffin (1)

Whole grain pita or tortilla (1)

GRAINS

Barley (½ cup cooked)

Brown or wild rice (½ cup cooked)

Cereal, high-fiber, low sugar (1 cup)

Oats, steel-cut (¼ cup dry) or old-fashioned rolled oats (½ cup dry)

Quinoa (½ cup cooked)

Whole grain couscous (½–1 cup cooked)

Whole grain pasta (½–1 cup cooked)

DAIRY & DAIRY SUBSTITUTES

Almond milk, unsweetened (1 cup)

Fat-free milk (1 cup)

Fat-free or part-skim ricotta cheese (½ cup)

Low-fat or reduced-fat cheeses

(¼ c grated or 1 oz)

Nonfat or low-fat regular yogurt, fruit-flavored or plain (6–8 oz)

Reduced-fat string cheese (1–2 pieces)

(continued)

Phase 3 Mile-High Metabolism Foods—*Continued*

REINFORCE CARBOHYDRATES—Continued

BEANS & STARCHY VEGETABLES

Beans (½ cup whole;
⅓ cup fat-free refried)

Baked potato (1 medium, 6–8 oz)

Corn (1 cup or 1 medium ear)

Edamame (½ cup shelled)

Peas (1 cup)

Pumpkin (1 cup mashed)

Sweet potato (4 oz, ½ cup mashed)

Winter squash (4 oz, ½ cup mashed)

VEGETABLE CARBOHYDRATES

These should be your only carb source at three meals or snacks a day.
However, you can have as much and as many of them as you like. You can
also have them in addition to Reinforce Carbs at any meal.

Artichoke

Asparagus

Beets

Broccoli

Brussels sprouts

Cabbage and Chinese cabbage
(such as bok choy)

Carrots

Cauliflower

Celery

Cucumbers

Dark leafy greens (collards, kale,
spinach, Swiss chard)

Eggplant

Fennel

Green beans

Mushrooms

Onions, scallions

Parsnips

Peppers, sweet and hot

Salad greens—all varieties

Summer squash

Tomato and tomato sauce

Turnips and rutabagas

Zucchini

ONLY THE HEALTHIEST FATS

Include fat in two meals or snacks per day.

NUTS

Almond butter (1 Tbsp)

Almonds (15–18)

Peanut butter (1 Tbsp)

Pistachios (25)

Walnuts (8–9 halves)

Oils

Canola oil (1 Tbsp)	Olive oil (1 Tbsp)

Other

Avocado (⅓ medium)	Olives (10 small, 5 medium/large)
Hummus (¼ cup)	

HOW TO MOVE

In phase 3, your goal is to maintain the activity level you reached at the end of phase 2—either 70 minutes of planned activity 6 days per week or 35 minutes of planned activity with a minimum of 7,000 lifestyle steps per day 6 days a week. Now is a good time to review all that you've achieved. Has physical activity become a part of your life? Do you have more energy now that you are active? Are you focusing on the positive benefits of movement? Have you discovered how to fit 70 minutes of movement into the 1,440 minutes of your day? Have you developed routines and rituals that make you confident you can continue to meet your movement goals forever? If the answers to these questions are yes, congratulations. You're on the road to the state of slim. If you answer no to any of them, it's time to make some changes. If you don't like the activities you're doing, experiment with something different. You have many options. If timing is your issue, try being active at different times of day. Would you benefit from joining a gym, YMCA, or fitness club or by considering a personal trainer or a wellness coach? We don't want you to reverse all the progress you've worked so hard to achieve.

THINK THIN

You're in the home stretch! It's time to solidify your Colorado Mind-Set to accompany your Mile-High Metabolism and celebrate your achievements!

1. **REVAMP YOUR LIST OF WHYS.** By now, you should have a few whys that relate to your purpose and come from internal motivation. Go over your list and add or delete whys. Keep it up to date. Use it to remind yourself why sticking to the Colorado Diet is worthwhile.

2. **FOCUS ON THE NEW YOU AND YOUR NEW LIFE.** You have the opportunity to reinvent yourself as someone who lives and values a healthy lifestyle, to make new friends who also value this way of living, and to become an optimist. We want you to continue your ritual of listing what you are grateful for every day. But now we also want you to start a list of all the good things that have happened to you *because of* your new smarter eating strategy, your increase in activity, and your weight loss. As we mentioned in Chapter 3, patients who see the positive in their new lifestyle do much better than the ones who constantly talk about how bad or hard the new path is. You—and only you—have the power to determine how you perceive your own reality. It's only horrible if you think it's horrible.

3. **DEVELOP SPECIAL-OCCASION ROUTINES AND RITUALS.** At this point, you're probably comfortable following the Colorado Diet at home, but you may feel shaky when

you're away from your normal environment. Restaurants are a particular stumbling block for most people, so we ask you to come up with one restaurant routine or ritual that will help you in the weeks ahead. For example, one of Holly's routines is to always send the bread basket back. Other good options: Start with salad even before you order the rest of your meal, or always share your entrée or cut it in half.

Work environments and holidays are other tough situations that can push you off track. During phase 3, there likely will be a holiday or special occasion, so develop a ritual to handle it. Even if nothing pops up, think of a strategy you can use later. For instance, many cities host a 5-K or 10-K turkey trot on Thanksgiving morning. Why not make attending it a family ritual? This is a triple win. You get to be active, spend quality time with your family, and associate with other active people.

Travel is another potential plan buster. When you're logging business miles, maybe you end up eating in your car. Perhaps you have trouble getting in your 70 minutes of walking on those overnight business trips. Maybe you succumb to the lure of the doughnut during a morning meeting. Think about your challenges and come up with a ritual to get you through tough situations.

4.   **EXPAND YOUR ACTIVE SOCIAL NETWORK.** While it's true that Colorado has an athletic population, such people exist in every state, city, and town. Reaching beyond your usual group of companions to find new, active friendships is invaluable: Being around people who value movement

means you have a higher chance of being active, too. That's exactly what you want.

Don't be afraid to ask people to join you. There are countless ways to reach out to people who have common healthy lifestyle interests. Start a walking club in your neighborhood or at work. Initiate a healthy cooking or dining club in which you go to healthy restaurants. Many neighborhoods hold progressive dinners as a way to build relationships with neighbors; make yours health centered. If you own a dog, find a friend who has one as well and begin walking your pets together. Take dance lessons. If you like aquatic sports, check into joining a masters swimming team. Look into volunteer opportunities that allow you to share what you have learned about living a healthy lifestyle with others. Find something healthy that taps into your passion, then go for it. See Resources on page 227 for more suggestions.

WHAT'S NEXT?

At the end of phase 3, you have a choice: Stick with phase 3 for an additional 6 weeks and lose more weight, or move into the Mile-High Metabolism Forever stage (Chapter 9) and maintain your new slender body. Either way, remember to keep moving forward in expanding your new mind-set and building your supportive environment, both physically and socially.

FINDING INNER MOTIVATION

Nora never had a weight problem until two pregnancies and a bout with thyroid cancer threw her metabolism out of whack. As the Cincinnati resident struggled to manage life with a new job and two young children, she began rewarding herself with food—mostly baked goods and starchy pasta. Before long, she was carrying 40 extra pounds on her 5-foot-6-inch frame. She felt "bulky" and could hardly stand to look at herself in the mirror. Her desire to change came from within. Seeing her image reflected, she recalls, "I said to myself, 'Is this who you are?' I couldn't get comfortable with that thought." So she made a commitment to herself that she would lose the extra weight. She did it mostly by planning her meals in advance. She eliminated the sugary sweets and baked goods from her home and surrounded herself with good food choices. Knowing that she sometimes has the urge to snack, she makes sure she always keeps low-calorie choices within reach, like 100-calorie bagel thins. She eats breakfast every morning, and she makes a plan to navigate tricky food situations. If she's attending a meeting where high-calorie snacks or hors d'oeuvres will be served, she'll eat a bowl of hearty soup beforehand to ensure she arrives with a full stomach. She's careful and thoughtful during the week, but on weekends she allows herself a couple of indulgence meals. She never overdoes it, but she enjoys a glass or two of wine with dinner and a steak or a sweet now and again, too. Now 58, Nora has maintained a weight loss of 40 pounds for 17 years. She doesn't feel deprived—she feels empowered and healthy.

A Mile-High
Metabolism—Forever

CONGRATULATIONS. YOU'VE REACHED A major milestone. You've lost weight and developed a metabolism that works for, rather than against, you. You've got more energy and very likely more confidence. You're in the state of slim, and you're now set to live a lean and healthy lifestyle for good.

So now what? At this point in your journey, you have a choice to make. You can switch over to the Colorado lifestyle we describe in this chapter, which represents the forever part of the Colorado Diet. Or, if you still have weight to lose, you can stay in phase 3 for up to 6 more weeks. This would make a total of 22 weeks—or 5 months—of weight loss. After that, though, you should switch to the Colorado lifestyle before trying to lose more weight (see why in the next section). What you *can't* do is go back to the way you were eating and what you were doing before you began this journey. If you return to your old habits, you'll revert to your old body and your old you. Celebrate your accomplishments—but also make a decision to sustain the new body and life you've created.

WHY CAN'T I JUST KEEP ON LOSING WEIGHT?

The fact is, people do not lose weight forever. We're just not wired that way. In the majority of the studies we've done, weight loss slows over time and usually stops by 5 or 6 months. One reason for this is that as you become slimmer, your body requires less and less energy, so you have to eat less and less to keep the weight loss going. Second, as we have explained, the longer we restrict our calories, the more our brains intensify hunger signals to try to get us to eat. Our research shows that while people are very compliant with diet changes initially, they become less compliant over time. We've seen that the loss of momentum tends to make people feel unsuccessful in spite of the fact that they're still following the diet. Oftentimes, people feel as though the program is no longer working, and they give up. The result: The weight just comes back.

But there is a way to trick your body: Give it a break. Losing some weight, then allowing your body to get used to keeping it off before trying to lose more, makes much more biological sense than repeating cycles of loss and regain. Think of losing weight in stages—20 to 40 pounds at a time. We know weight loss and weight-loss maintenance are different animals, and you need to develop a skill set for both to achieve long-term success.

Spend 3 months on this maintenance phase to allow your body to adjust to your new, slimmer shape. After 3 months, you'll have overridden your body's resistance to additional weight loss, and you can begin the Colorado Diet again to melt away more pounds. As long as you've been maintaining your 70 minutes of activity 6 days a week, you can restart the diet on phase 2 or 3. If you've let your activity slip, we suggest you repeat all three phases.

THE COLORADO LIFESTYLE: FIVE STEPS TO PERMANENTLY LEAN

We know what lean and healthy forever looks like, because we've seen it among people in the National Weight Control Registry (NWCR). And the way they live looks very much like the way most Coloradans live.

Using our research with the NWCR and our Colorado experience, we have developed a five-step plan to keep you at your new body weight. It will allow you to maintain your new, slimmer physique while eating a satisfying amount of food. No food restriction— just smart eating. As you follow these five steps, don't forget to continue to fine-tune your Colorado Mind-Set. Regularly think about why you want to stay at your new healthy weight. Focus on the positives and expect your new lifestyle to be great. Continue to develop habits, routines, and rituals—especially for being active. Finally, make sure you are surrounded by a healthy physical environment and by friends and family who value a healthy lifestyle and who support you.

1 / Keep Your Activity Level High

If we were in Las Vegas betting on the odds of your long-term success, we'd place our bet according to how consistent you've been with your physical activity plan. It's the biggest predictor of long-term weight loss, hands down. Think of physical activity like a medication for your

TOTAL TRANSFORMATION

When Donielle came to our clinic, she was ready for a change. She was 5 foot 2, and her weight had recently hit 186 pounds. "It made me sad to look at myself. Nothing fit me, and my knees hurt all the time," she recalls. Holly asked her to make a list of goals. Number one was to be able to fit into a cute skirt she had in her closet that she could no longer zip up. She knew she had to prioritize exercise, something that had been challenging for her in the past. So this time she decided to enlist her family's help. Her husband began walking with her regularly, and they set up a treadmill and an exercise bike in front of the TV so that they could exercise together while they watched their favorite shows. Workout time became family time. Even her youngest daughter took part—on her rocking horse.

Donielle lost 5 pounds her first week on the Colorado Diet. As she started walking and eventually running, she noticed her appetite coming into balance with her activity level. By the end of phase 3, she had lost 42 pounds.

Although she could zip up that skirt, she discovered an even greater payoff: She actually enjoyed exercise. "I never saw myself as weight. Everyone wants a pill to increase their metabolism, but you have something better—a Mile-High Metabolism—and it's more potent than any pill. Just as you wouldn't expect your medication to work if you didn't take it, you can't expect to keep a Mile-High Metabolism if you skip your recommended dose of physical activity.

a runner when I started this process, but now I love it. I see running not as a chore but as something that is a big part of my life. It's weird how it changed for me," she notes. Recently, she finished a 5-K race. "It felt like such an accomplishment! Much more so than fitting into the skirt," she says. "It took mental drive, and it felt really good inside."

To maintain her Colorado lifestyle, she set a new goal of running a half-marathon and joined a running group. While she would like to lose a few more pounds in the future, she has set a "take-action" weight of 145 pounds, and she weighs herself at least every other day. She's come to appreciate the flavor of her new, healthy diet. "Looking back, I enjoy what I eat so much more now than when I weighed 186 pounds," Donielle observes. To top things off, she got some good news at her annual physical: Her total cholesterol went from 215 to 133, her HDL or good cholesterol increased from 30 to 41, her LDL (bad) cholesterol reached an impressive low of 75, and her triglycerides plummeted from 250 to 88. "This was just the cherry on top of the cake for me," she says. "I feel like I've reinvented myself and there is more good stuff to come."

2 / Eat High-Quality Foods—Most of the Time

No more lists of foods. No more measuring your portions. After you complete phase 3, your metabolism has adjusted to the point where you can eat a broader, less-restrictive range of foods. Because you're keeping your activity high, you can continue to enjoy occasional indulgence foods and indulgence meals. However, this doesn't mean you can return to your old eating habits. You must still eat smart— the majority of your diet should consist of the high-quality foods you've been eating these past 16 weeks. You don't want your drain to become clogged again!

During phases 1 through 3, you probably discovered meals that were easy to prepare and especially satisfying. Make these your go-to meals. Keep the ingredients for them readily available and continue to use your environment to support your new lifestyle. If you know you always overeat potato chips, don't keep them in your house. Rather, enjoy a reasonable portion of chips at a restaurant or at a friend's party. A good strategy is to follow what's known as the 80/20 rule: Eat a healthful diet 80 percent of the time and give yourself permission to eat however you like 20 percent of the time.

3 / Monitor Your Weight

You need to weigh yourself every day—at the same time, on the same scale. This should become a habit that you continue for the rest of your life. Just as a person with diabetes needs to check his or her blood sugar, you'll need to monitor your weight. Even NWCR participants who have been lean for decades report that they weigh themselves regularly. One recently said, "How will I know I'm gaining weight unless I step on the scale?"

We're aware that some experts recommend getting rid of the

scale on the theory that small gains will just make you crazy. We disagree. You may think you can detect weight gain by noticing how your clothes fit, but the scale is better. It's black and white. Your jeans may be *kinda* tight, but you do not *kinda* weigh 150 pounds. You need this objective information for long-term success.

4 / Set a "Take-Action" Weight

The scale is a valuable tool that provides useful information—if you know what to do with it. That's where your take-action weight comes in. Even if you faithfully adhere to steps 1 through 3, it's almost inevitable that you will have times when you regain some of your weight. This might be during an illness, a holiday or vacation, a very stressful life event, a job change, or even just when things get really busy. If you decide ahead of time that you will reexamine your eating and exercise when the scale reads 3 to 5 pounds over the weight you'd like to maintain, you can keep 5 pounds from becoming 15. For example, if you weigh 175 pounds at the end of phase 3 and want to maintain this weight, you need to take action if the scale creeps up to 178 to 180 pounds. However, don't worry if your weight fluctuates from day to day—as long as it stays below your take-action weight.

Take this number seriously. Write it down on a piece of paper and stick it to your scale or on the bathroom mirror, where you see it every day. When you hit your take-action weight, allow yourself no excuses—no thinking "it's just water weight," "it's hormonal," or "I'll deal with it later." Your take-action weight means you take action *period,* regardless of the reason your weight might be up.

What action should you take? It depends. If you've let your daily activity plan slip, get yourself back on the program (reread Chapter 4). If you're meeting your daily physical activity goal, then you'll need to modify your diet. The easiest way to do this is to go back to phase 1 or 2 of the Colorado Diet. Most people find it reassuring to return to a more structured eating plan when they start gaining weight. Pay attention to portions and limit indulgence meals to no more than one per week. Increase the number of vegetable carbohydrate sources and eat fewer carbs. It's okay to use trial and error. Find out what works for you and incorporate this into your take-action plan. Lose the 3 to 5 pounds and revert to the Colorado lifestyle.

5 / Be a Role Model

In medical school, Holly discovered that the best way to really learn something is to teach it to someone else. Now that you understand what it takes to lose weight and keep it off, you can help others. We're not asking you to become preachy about it, but we'd like you to be open to sharing what you've learned with a family member or coworker who wants to shed pounds or become healthier. We bet you have many friends who also struggle with weight. As you help guide others, it will reinforce your own commitment.

Perhaps, though, your actions can have the greatest influence on your children. The lifestyle you are living now is the best one for your children's health, regardless of whether they have a weight problem. By following the Colorado lifestyle, you are teaching them by example the importance of healthy eating and activity—and showing them that it can be fun. You can even get involved in your children's school. Most schools are working hard to create healthier environments for students. (See Resources on page 227 for information on a program called 5th Gear Kids that we've implemented in

LONG-TERM SUCCESS

Mary is one of the first members of the National Weight Control Registry—she lost 50 pounds nearly 40 years ago. In her late twenties, she found herself at 155 pounds. That was a lot to carry on her 5-foot frame, but the discomfort of being overweight wasn't what motivated her to slim down. Rather, her biggest why was connected to her two young daughters. "I didn't want them to live with the stigma of having a fat mom," she says. She initially lost weight with a low-carb diet, but she's kept it off all these years by following the Colorado lifestyle.

Today, Mary's diet centers on healthful, enjoyable foods that make her feel satisfied instead of deprived—just as it did back then. She's also made exercise an essential part of her day and figured out how to fit it into her life. Always an early riser, she began walking 4 miles in the mornings around her neighborhood, and if she wanted to catch up with a friend, she suggested a walk in the park instead of meeting for lunch—two rituals she's continued to this day. She even uses walking to enrich family time: Whenever her now-grown daughters visit, they join her on her morning walks.

Her self-esteem evolved as her body changed. Once shy and hesitant, she became more and more outgoing as her confidence improved. Now, at age 66, Mary is a poised, outgoing instructor in our weight-loss clinic, helping other people discover the Colorado lifestyle.

some Denver-area schools to teach fifth graders about healthy living. It might be of interest to schools in your community.)

ENJOY THE NEW YOU

The Colorado lifestyle is no longer a goal, it's simply the way you live. Gone are your days of counting calories and still having trouble with your weight. Eating smart is still a priority, but you can have real foods, enjoy meals out with friends without any guilt, and maintain your Mile-High Metabolism. Your taste buds have adjusted, and, if you're like many of our patients, old favorites with fat or sugar don't taste as good as they used to. You've come to prefer your new way of eating. Similarly, you now feel so energized and healthy, you wouldn't dream of living without regular physical activity. But perhaps the biggest transformation has happened in your mind. You've learned to focus on the positive and expect success. You've developed a strong sense of purpose and adopted habits, routines, and rituals that support the values that matter to you most. You are no longer someone who struggles to live healthfully; you think of yourself as a thin person. You've worked hard to get here, so take a minute to savor your success. Have fun with the new you. Then reinforce your commitment to living in the state of slim for good.

The Colorado Diet Recipes

CHAPTER 10

THE COLORADO DIET IS all about simple, fresh, and flavorful food. It's also about eating smarter. We like to think of it as the "mile-high flavor" diet, the perfect way to fuel your Mile-High Metabolism. We didn't develop a day-by-day eating plan—on day 1 eat this, on day 2 eat that—because we want you to have maximum flexibility on the Colorado Diet. (However, if you want suggestions for exactly what to eat, you can look at our sample daily menus in Appendix I on page 231.) Think of these recipes as ideas to help you get started. They're proof that by using fresh ingredients and flavor boosters like herbs and spices, you can have an amazing culinary experience and still fuel your Mile-High Metabolism while losing weight.

We've developed recipes for all three phases and have noted which phase they're appropriate for. Phase 1–friendly recipes are made with only phase 1 foods, but they can and should also be eaten in phases 2 and 3. And of course, phase 2 recipes can be served in phase 3 as well.

You may notice in some of our recipes that two or even three sources of protein or carbohydrates are listed as ingredients. The recipes have been designed so that when you eat one serving of the recipe you are getting the equivalent of one serving of a lean protein and one serving of a carbohydrate. In addition, in some of the recipes, a small amount of oil is used; if it accounts for 1 teaspoon or less of oil per serving, it doesn't count toward your daily fat servings.

BUILDING FLAVOR

If you're used to eating dishes loaded with fat, sugar, and salt, your taste buds will notice the change once you switch to the Colorado Diet. However, we're sure you've dined at a nice restaurant somewhere and had a dish that was bursting with flavor—not because it was high in fat, sugar, or salt, but thanks to the fresh ingredients, herbs, and spices it contained.

So how do you take a boneless, skinless chicken breast and make it tasty without using a ton of fat? What about a fillet of fish? Or a nice piece of lean pork? These lean protein foods are the foundation of the Colorado Diet. Lean meats, by definition, don't contain much fat, which would normally impart a lot of flavor. But there are several ways to get around that.

The first is to buy the freshest meat or fish available. (In some parts of the country, though, frozen fish may be your only choice.) Use herbs, spices, onions, garlic, and other seasonings to add flavor.

The next key is to avoid overcooking. Aim for medium-rare beef or pork (or, in the case of poultry, cook just until the juices run clear and the pink has just disappeared); beyond that stage, lean meat becomes tough and tasteless. Overcooking can destroy a perfectly tasty vegetable, too. Chances are that people who don't like vegetables (and maybe you are one of them) have suffered through too many servings of mushy broccoli, drab green beans, and slimy spinach. Vegetables are so much more flavorful when you cook them so they retain their natural bright colors and they're tender with a slight crispness.

Finally, there are endless ways to dress up lean proteins or vegetables without smothering the food in butter. These include spice rubs for meat and fish, herbs, salsa, low-sugar juice, vinegars, and low-fat condiments like mustard. We give you examples of these techniques in our phase 1 recipes.

Many of the following recipes suggest using fresh herbs, and most of these are commonly available at your local grocery. Kept in a sealed bag with a paper towel to control moisture, fresh herbs can last a week in the refrigerator. Some stores sell small potted herb plants, like basil, thyme, or rosemary, that you can keep on a window shelf or back porch. This is the gift that keeps on giving, as trimming off the leaves to use in your cooking stimulates the plant to grow more!

Sometimes, however, you don't have access to fresh herbs, and it's absolutely acceptable to use dried versions that are readily available at the grocery. Many of our soup recipes, for example, call for dried herbs because their flavor better withstands prolonged cooking than fresh. A good rule of thumb is to use about one-third as much of a dried herb as you would the fresh. However, dried herbs don't last forever. They lose their pizzazz over time and can actually turn bitter. Check the expiration date on the package. To make sure your dried herbs and spices don't go out of date, don't buy them in giant containers like the ones sold at club stores.

Breakfast

Chocolate Cheesecake Muffins

Bake a batch on the weekend and freeze in small resealable plastic bags (2 muffins per bag). They are low in fat and sugar and pack a punch of protein and phase I Reignite carbohydrate to get you going. Eat them for breakfast or after a workout or when you want something a little sweet. They are one of our patients' favorite go-to meals.

1 cup old-fashioned rolled oats (not quick-cooking)
½ cup stevia (baking formulation)
2 scoops chocolate protein powder
1 tablespoon fat-free cheesecake pudding mix
1 tablespoon unsweetened cocoa powder
1 teaspoon baking powder
1 teaspoon baking soda
1 cup liquid egg whites
½ cup nonfat plain Greek yogurt

Preheat the oven to 350°F. Coat 12 cups of a muffin pan with cooking spray (see Tip).

In a blender, grind the oats to a flourlike consistency.

In a large bowl, whisk together the ground oats, stevia, protein powder, pudding mix, cocoa, baking powder, and baking soda. Pour in the egg whites and yogurt and whisk until smooth. Divide the batter evenly among the muffin cups.

Bake until a wooden pick inserted in a muffin comes out clean, 15 to 20 minutes. Eat while still warm or freeze for later.

Makes 12 muffins/6 servings
1 serving = 1 protein & 1 Reignite carbohydrate

Tip: *If you are going to use liners in the muffin pan, they need to be foil liners with the paper removed. Unlike muffins made with wheat flour, oat flour will stick to paper liners and give you a huge headache. Even the foil liners should be coated with cooking spray!*

Cinnamon-Pumpkin Protein Pancakes

These pancakes have the perfect carbohydrate-protein combination to get your day going. Add I tablespoon of low-sugar jelly or sugar-free syrup as a topping. Alternatively, mix a small amount of PB2 in a bowl and spread it between 2 pancakes for a mock peanut butter sandwich. The pancakes are most delicious freshly made and warm, but you can freeze them and reheat, too.

1½ cups old-fashioned rolled oats (not quick-cooking)
2 scoops vanilla protein powder
I tablespoon stevia (baking formulation)
1½ teaspoons baking powder
1½ teaspoons ground cinnamon
1½ cups liquid egg whites
¼ cup canned unsweetened pumpkin puree

In a blender or food processor, grind the oats to a flourlike consistency. Transfer to a bowl and whisk in the protein powder, stevia, baking powder, and cinnamon. Whisk in the egg whites and pumpkin until smooth.

Preheat a griddle or skillet. Coat with cooking spray. Pour the batter onto the griddle or skillet in 3"-diameter rounds. Cook for about 3 minutes on one side and then flip to cook the other side.

Makes 20 (2" to 3") pancakes/5 servings
I serving = I protein & I Reignite carbohydrate

PHASE I FRIENDLY
_____
REIGNITE YOUR METABOLISM
_____
WEEKS 1–2

Egg-White Omelet with Fresh Veggies

In phase 3, add fat-free or low-fat cheese when you add the veggies. You can also add 2 tablespoons of salsa when you add the veggies.

½ cup chopped onion
½ cup sliced mushrooms
½ cup diced green bell pepper
½ cup diced red bell pepper
1 cup egg whites or pasteurized egg whites
Salt and freshly ground black pepper

Coat a 10" nonstick skillet with olive oil spray and heat over medium heat. Add the onion, mushrooms, and bell peppers and cook, stirring occasionally, until tender, about 10 minutes. Transfer to a plate.

Respray the pan with olive oil and place back over medium heat. Add the egg whites and season with salt and pepper to taste. Continue cooking, lifting the edges with a large spatula as the egg whites start to set and tipping the pan to allow the uncooked whites to run underneath. Cook for 2 to 3 minutes, or until the eggs are set.

With the spatula, flip the omelet over in the pan. Spoon the cooked veggies over half the omelet and fold the omelet over the veggies. Cook for 1 minute.

Makes 1 serving
1 serving = 1 protein & 1 vegetable carbohydrate

PHASE 2 FRIENDLY
REBUILD YOUR METABOLISM
WEEKS 3–8

Very Berry Energizing Oatmeal

This oatmeal is a great easy way to get your protein in to start your day. You can make several variations of this recipe by using other flavors of protein powder, such as chocolate, choosing different fresh fruits, or even adding in a serving of peanut or almond butter when you are in phase 3. Omit the fruit and it will fit in as a phase 1–friendly recipe. You can add 1 tablespoon of sugar-free jam or jelly in phase 1 for a little fruit flavor.

1 cup water
½ cup old-fashioned rolled oats (not quick-cooking)
Dash of salt (optional)
1 scoop vanilla protein powder
½ cup blueberries or strawberries
Stevia or sugar substitute to taste (optional)

In a medium saucepan, combine the almond milk or water, oats, and salt (if using). Bring to a boil and cook over medium heat, stirring occasionally, for 5 to 6 minutes. Remove from the heat and, while the mixture is still creamy with some liquid remaining, quickly stir in the protein powder. Transfer to a bowl and allow to cool slightly. Top with fresh berries. Sprinkle stevia or a sugar substitute on top, if desired, for added sweetness.

Makes 1 serving
1 serving = 1 protein & 1 Rebuild carbohydrate

PHASE 3 FRIENDLY

REINFORCE YOUR METABOLISM

WEEKS 9–16

Lemon–Chia Seed Muffins

The lemon yogurt makes this a phase 3 recipe. You can have fun with this recipe by using blueberry or other flavors of nonfat yogurt, trying other extracts, and changing the flavor of the protein powder. Be creative and come up with your own muffin types.

I cup old-fashioned rolled oats (not quick-cooking)
½ cup stevia (baking formulation)
2 scoops vanilla protein powder
I tablespoon chia seeds
I teaspoon baking soda
I teaspoon baking powder
I cup liquid egg whites
6 ounces nonfat lemon-flavored yogurt
I teaspoon lemon extract

Preheat the oven to 350°F. Coat 12 cups of a muffin pan with cooking spray (see Tip on page 184).

In a blender, grind the oats to a flourlike consistency.

In a large bowl, combine the ground oats, stevia, protein powder, chia seeds, baking soda, and baking powder. Pour in the egg whites, yogurt, and extract and whisk until smooth.

(continued)

Divide the batter evenly among the muffin cups. Bake until a wooden pick inserted in the center of a muffin comes out clean, 15 to 20 minutes. Eat while still warm or refrigerate (3 days) or freeze (longer term) for later.

Makes 12 muffins/6 servings
1 serving = 1 protein & 1 Reinforce carbohydrate

Tip: *If you want to line the muffin pan, choose foil liners with the paper removed. Unlike muffins made with wheat flour, oat flour will stick to paper liners and give you a huge headache. Even the foil liners should be coated with cooking spray!*

PHASE 3 FRIENDLY
REINFORCE YOUR METABOLISM
WEEKS 9–16

Sausage and Egg Mile-High Muffin

Egg whites also cook very well in the microwave. Coat a small micro-waveable bowl or large mug with cooking spray, add the egg whites and hot sauce, microwave for 1 minute, stir gently, and microwave for 30 more seconds or until set. Allow to cool slightly.

1 lean turkey sausage patty, usually about 1½ ounces or 60 calories
3 egg whites or 1 whole egg + 1 egg white
1 slice reduced-fat or fat-free American or Cheddar cheese
1 whole grain English muffin or bagel thin, split and toasted
Hot sauce (optional)

Coat a small nonstick skillet with cooking spray. Add the sausage patty and heat. Place the patty on a plate. Add the egg whites or egg to the skillet. Cook for 1 to 2 minutes, or until the egg whites set in the middle and the bottom starts to brown. Flip the egg whites or egg. Cook for 1 minute, or until completely set.

Place the cheese on the bottom half of the muffin or bagel thin, followed by the egg, hot sauce (if using), and ham or sausage patty. Top with the other half of the muffin or bagel thin.

Makes 1 serving
1 serving = 1 protein & 1 Reinforce carbohydrate

Main Dishes

Baked Salmon with Mustard Dill Sauce

This dish pairs well with asparagus or wilted spinach in phase 1. In phase 2, you can serve it with brown rice and scallions. The mustard sauce can be made the day before and kept covered in the refrigerator. And don't worry about the brandy in the sauce; the alcohol cooks off, and you wouldn't know there was brandy in it.

2 pounds skin-on salmon fillet (see Tip)
¼ cup yellow mustard
¼ cup brown mustard
2 tablespoons reduced-sodium soy sauce
2 tablespoons brandy
1½ teaspoons dried dillweed

Preheat the oven to 350°F. Take the fish out of the refrigerator and allow to warm to room temperature. Line a baking sheet with foil.

Rinse the salmon under cold water and pat dry with paper towels. Place the fish skin-side down on the foil.

In a bowl, whisk together the yellow and brown mustards, soy, brandy, and dill. Using a spoon, cover the fish with the mustard sauce, making sure that no pink is showing.

Bake until the flesh loses its translucency and is a uniform light pink (check the flesh in the thickest part of the fillet), 12 to 18 minutes (depending on the fillet's thickness). Serve hot.

Makes 6 to 8 servings
I serving = I protein & I fat

Tip: *You can make this recipe with individual 4- to 5-ounce salmon fillets; they will just take less time to cook.*

Chicken Tenders with Spicy Summer Squash

Spices can take a routine vegetable and make it taste fabulous. Even if you're not a vegetable lover at this point—say you're trying to make some different veggies—experiment with spices. As you progress through the steps of the Colorado Diet, your taste buds will change. Give spices a try—the results might surprise you.

I pound chicken breast tenders
Salt and freshly ground black pepper
Cajun or Creole seasoning blend (or another spicy seasoning mix of
    your choice)
2 large yellow summer squash, peeled and cut crosswise into ½"-thick
    slices
I large zucchini, peeled and cut crosswise into ½"-thick slices
I tablespoon olive oil (optional)

Coat a large nonstick skillet with cooking spray or olive oil spray and place over medium heat. Sprinkle the chicken with salt and pepper. Place the chicken in the skillet and cook, turning once, or until browned on both sides and no longer pink in the center, about 10 minutes. Transfer to a plate.

Sprinkle the seasoning mix on both sides of the squash and zucchini slices. Increase the heat under the skillet to high and add the vegetables (you can add the olive oil to help sauté if you have not had your good fats for the day). Cook, flipping frequently, until tender, about 5 minutes. Serve the squash alongside the chicken.

Makes 4 servings

1 serving = 1 protein & 1 vegetable carbohydrate
and 1 fat (if oil is used)

PHASE I FRIENDLY

REIGNITE YOUR METABOLISM

WEEKS 1–2

Herbed Chicken Roll-Ups with Spinach and Roasted Red Pepper

You can buy jarred roasted red peppers in the supermarket or roast your own. If you use store-bought peppers, be sure to wash them thoroughly under cold water to rinse off the packing brine.

2 boneless, skinless chicken breast cutlets (4–5 ounces each),
    trimmed of any external fat

1 clove garlic, halved

1 teaspoon dried basil

1 teaspoon dried oregano

1 teaspoon dried thyme

Pinch of salt

Pinch of freshly ground black pepper

3 ounces fresh spinach

1 roasted red pepper, halved

2 teaspoons olive oil

Preheat the oven to 350°F.

Cover a cutting board with a sheet of plastic wrap. Put a chicken breast on the board and cover with a second sheet of plastic wrap. Pound the chicken breast with a meat hammer or the flat side of a small skillet until it is about ¼" thick. Repeat with the second chicken breast.

Rub the cut garlic over 1 side of each chicken breast. This will be the inside when you roll it up. In a small bowl, mix together the basil, oregano, thyme, and salt and pepper. Using half of the mixture, dust the inside surface of each chicken breast. Cover each chicken breast with a layer of spinach leaves. Then lay one-half of the roasted red pepper over the spinach on each breast. Starting at 1 end, tightly roll up each breast with the grain, taking care not to push out the spinach and pepper filling as you roll. To hold the roll together, you can either tie it with 1 or 2 pieces of kitchen twine or close the end with toothpicks. Using 1 teaspoon of the oil, rub the outsides of the rolls, then sprinkle evenly with the remaining herb mixture.

In a nonstick ovenproof skillet, heat the remaining 1 teaspoon oil over medium-high heat. When the oil is hot, place the rolls in the pan and cook, turning, 3 to 4 minutes, or for until the outside begins to show a light golden brown.

Place the pan in the oven and cook until the chicken is cooked through, 10 to 12 minutes.

To serve, slice the rolls crosswise to expose the colorful spinach and pepper insides and overlap them on plates. Be sure to remove the toothpicks or twine before serving.

Makes 2 servings
1 serving = 1 protein & 1 vegetable carbohydrate

Southwestern Chicken with Cilantro Cream Dipping Sauce

Serve the chicken skewers with the dipping sauce and a vegetable of your choice. In phase 1, try it with grilled or roasted asparagus, broccoli, or cauliflower.

¼ cup old-fashioned rolled oats (not quick-cooking)
2 tablespoons chili powder
½ teaspoon freshly ground black pepper
¼ teaspoon salt
¼ teaspoon ground red pepper
½ cup liquid egg whites
1 pound chicken breast tenders
Cilantro Cream Dipping Sauce (recipe follows)

Soak 4 wooden skewers in water for 30 minutes.

Preheat the oven to 400°F. Coat a baking sheet with cooking spray or olive oil spray.

In a blender, grind the oats to a flourlike consistency.

In a shallow dish, combine the ground oats, chili powder, black pepper, salt, and ground red pepper. Place the egg whites in a second dish. Dip the chicken tenders in the egg whites and then roll in the oat mixture. Thread the tenders onto the skewers.

Place the skewers on the baking sheet and bake until no longer pink, usually 8 to 10 minutes. If you want them to be crispy, you can broil them for the last few minutes, but watch them carefully so they don't burn.

Serve with the dipping sauce.

Makes 4 servings
I serving = I protein (including ¼ cup dipping sauce)

Cilantro Cream Dipping Sauce

You can make this tasty dip on its own and serve with crudités.

I cup (8 ounces) nonfat plain Greek yogurt
3 tablespoons chopped cilantro
Garlic salt or fresh garlic, minced

In a small bowl, stir together the yogurt, cilantro, and garlic salt or garlic to taste.

Makes about 1 cup
I cup = I protein

Crowd-Pleasing Slow-Cooker Pumpkin Chili

Make this in the fall for Sunday football. (The recipe is easily doubled for a crowd.) Start it early in the morning and your house will smell great by afternoon game time. Nobody ever suspects how healthy this chili really is. The pumpkin gives it a smooth texture and flavor even without any added fat or fatty cuts of meat. If you don't have a slow cooker, you can also do this on the stove in a heavy pot, like a Dutch oven. In phase 2 or 3 of the Colorado Diet, you can add kidney beans or your favorite bean to the recipe.

1 pound extra-lean ground beef or turkey breast
1 yellow onion, chopped
2 green bell peppers, chopped
1 fresh jalapeño chile pepper, seeded and chopped (optional),
    wear plastic gloves when handling
2 cloves garlic
1 can (15 ounces) unsweetened pumpkin puree
1 can (14 ounces) diced tomatoes
1 tablespoon chili powder (or more to taste)
2 teaspoons ground cumin
1 teaspoon salt
Freshly ground black pepper

Coat a large skillet with cooking spray and heat over medium heat Add the ground meat, breaking it up into pieces, and cook until browned, about 8 to 10 minutes.

In a 3- to 4-quart slow cooker, combine the ground meat, onion, bell peppers, jalapeño pepper (if using), garlic, pumpkin puree, tomatoes, chili powder, cumin, salt, black pepper to taste, and 1 cup water. Cover and cook on low heat for 6 to 7 hours, until the vegetables are tender. Stir to combine the ingredients, ladle into bowls, and serve hot.

Makes 4 servings
1 serving = 1 protein & 1 Reignite carbohydrate &
1 vegetable carbohydrate

Savory Pork Tacos with Wilted Arugula

Once you are in phase 3, you can use this same recipe and add reduced-fat cheese or reduced-fat sour cream just prior to serving.

2 boneless loin pork chops (½" thick, about 4 ounces each), trimmed of any visible fat
Low-Salt Spice Mix/Rub (page 224)
½ red onion, thinly sliced
1 large clove garlic, minced
1 jalapeño chile pepper, seeded and chopped (optional), wear plastic gloves when handling
6 ounces arugula
Handful of cherry tomatoes, halved
Pinch of salt
Pinch of freshly ground black pepper
6 corn tortillas (6" diameter, about 50 calories per tortilla)
2 tablespoons Simple Homemade Pico de Gallo (optional; page 222)

Sprinkle both sides of the pork evenly with some spice mix. Slice the seasoned chops diagonally across the grain into ¼"-wide strips.

Coat a large skillet with cooking spray and place over medium heat. Add the onion, garlic, and jalapeño pepper (if using) and cook for 1 minute. Add the pork strips and cook until the centers of the pork strips are still light pink, 1 to 2 minutes. You don't want to overcook the meat. Add the arugula and tomatoes to the pan and stir all the contents around until the arugula just begins to wilt. Immediately remove from the heat. Add the salt and pepper and toss.

Heat the tortillas in the microwave oven for 30 seconds or in an open pan on the stove over medium heat. You just want to warm them, not cook them so that they become too stiff. Fill the warm tortillas with the pork and vegetable mixture and serve. Top them off with pico de gallo, if you'd like, for a little spicy crunch.

Makes 2 servings

1 serving = 1 protein & 1 Rebuild carbohydrate &
1 vegetable carbohydrate

Fabulous Fish Tacos

You can serve these with Crunchy Mango Salsa (page 226) in phase 3. These tacos are also great with a little diced avocado for garnish.

I cup shredded red cabbage
I teaspoon cider vinegar
Salt and freshly ground black pepper
I teaspoon olive oil
½ cup diced red onion
2 fillets red snapper, halibut, or swordfish (4–5 ounces each),
    cut into I" chunks
6 corn tortillas (6" diameter, about 50 calories per tortilla)
½ cup diced red bell pepper
½ cup chopped fresh cilantro
½ lime, cut into wedges

In a bowl, toss the cabbage with the vinegar and a pinch of salt.

In a large nonstick skillet, heat the oil over medium-high heat. Add the onion and cook until soft, about 2 minutes, and set aside in a separate bowl. Season the fish with salt and pepper, place in the skillet, and cook over medium-high heat until just opaque, 3 to 4 minutes.

Warm the tortillas in a skillet or in the microwave oven with a paper towel on top and bottom. To assemble the tacos, divide the fish among the tortillas and top with the sautéed onion, cabbage, bell pepper, and cilantro. Serve with lime wedges.

Makes 2 servings

I serving = I protein & I Rebuild carbohydrate &
I vegetable carbohydrate

PHASE 2 FRIENDLY
REBUILD YOUR METABOLISM
WEEKS 3–8

Pan-Seared Salmon with Chile Oil and Wild Rice

In phase 3, this dish pairs well with the Crunchy Mango Salsa (page 226). The sauce offsets the spice from the chile oil and adds a soothing note.

2 skin-on salmon fillets (4–5 ounces each)
2 teaspoons chile oil (store-bought or homemade; recipe on page 200)
Salt and freshly ground black pepper
1 cup cooked wild rice
Chopped scallions

Preheat the oven to 350°F. Rinse the fillets under cold water and dry with a paper towel. Rub the chile oil on the flesh side of the salmon (not the skin side) and sprinkle with salt and pepper.

Heat a nonstick ovenproof skillet (or a regular skillet coated with cooking spray) over high heat. Add the fillets skin side up and cook for 30 seconds to 1 minute, or until a light brown crust appears. Flip the fillets over and cook skin side down for 30 to 45 seconds to crisp up the skin.

Transfer the skillet to the oven and bake until the flesh just loses its opacity and turns pink (do not overcook), about 10 minutes, depending on the thickness of the salmon.

Place the fish on a serving of rice and garnish with chopped scallions.

Makes 2 servings
1 serving = 1 protein & 1 Rebuild carbohydrate & 1 fat

Homemade Chile Oil

This beautiful red oil can be used to spice up salad dressing, as a rub for chicken or pork, or added to anything where you want a little zing. Stored in a cool, dark place, it will keep for 2 to 3 months.

½ cup canola or peanut oil
2 tablespoons red pepper flakes

In a small saucepan, heat the oil to 250°F (use a thermometer). Add the pepper flakes and stir well. Turn off the heat and let the pan sit at room temperature for at least 2 hours. Strain the mixture through a sieve and discard the pepper flakes.

Makes ½ cup
I tablespoon = I fat

PHASE 2 FRIENDLY
_____
REBUILD YOUR METABOLISM
_____
WEEKS 3–8

Pan-Sautéed Shrimp with Brown and Wild Rice Medley

If you've made a batch of the Brown and Wild Rice Medley ahead, this delicious dish can be ready in less than 20 minutes.

1 lemon
3 tablespoons chopped flat-leaf parsley
1½ teaspoons paprika
½ teaspoon red pepper flakes
3 dozen extra-jumbo (16/20 size) shrimp, peeled and deveined
Salt and freshly ground black pepper
3–4 tablespoons olive oil or Homemade Chile Oil (page 200)
Brown and Wild Rice Medley (page 211)

Grate the lemon peel to get 1 teaspoon of zest and juice the lemon. Set the juice aside. In a small bowl, mix together the lemon zest, parsley, paprika, and red pepper flakes.

Dry the shrimp on paper towels. Sprinkle the shrimp with salt and pepper. Toss the shrimp in the spice and lemon mixture to coat.

In a large skillet, heat the oil over medium-high heat. Working in batches, add the shrimp and sear in the oil until they just lose their translucency and turn light pink, about 2 minutes per side. Add the lemon juice and toss. Serve on a bed of the Brown and Wild Rice Medley.

Makes 4 servings
1 serving = 1 protein & 1 Rebuild carbohydrate & 1 fat

Spice-Rubbed Pork Tenderloin with Balsamic Reduction

This pairs well with a hearty vegetable like zucchini, or with Brown and Wild Rice Medley (page 211).

1 pork tenderloin (about 1 pound), trimmed of any fat and silver skin
1 teaspoon dried oregano
1 teaspoon dried thyme
1 teaspoon ground coriander
1 teaspoon ground cumin
1 teaspoon garlic powder
1 teaspoon freshly ground black pepper
1 tablespoon olive oil
½ cup balsamic vinegar

Preheat the oven to 400°F.

Rinse the pork and dry with paper towels. In a small bowl, mix together the oregano, thyme, coriander, cumin, garlic powder, and pepper. Coat the tenderloin with the herb and spice rub and place in the oven.

Preheat a large ovenproof skillet over medium-high heat. Add the olive oil and heat until it begins to shimmer. Add the pork and brown on all sides by turning with tongs, 8 to 10 minutes. Transfer the pork to the oven and bake until the center is uniformly pink, 15 to 20 minutes. Let rest for 5 minutes before slicing.

While the pork cooks, in a small saucepan, heat the vinegar over medium-high heat and cook until thick and syrupy and its volume is reduced by at least half, about 8 minutes.

Slice the pork across the grain into medallions and serve drizzled with the balsamic reduction.

Makes 4 servings
1 serving = 1 protein

Whole Wheat Pasta Puttanesca

Traditional puttanesca sauce has a ton of salt, using more anchovies, unsoaked capers, and lots more olives. This recipe cuts back on the salt but not the flavor. Serve with grilled boneless, skinless chicken breast cutlets or lean turkey sausage.

3 tablespoons capers
1 tablespoon olive oil
4 cloves garlic, minced
1 teaspoon anchovy paste
1 can (28 ounces) whole, peeled tomatoes
2 ounces kalamata olives, coarsely chopped
1 teaspoon dried oregano
1 teaspoon red pepper flakes
½ pound whole wheat pasta
3 tablespoons finely chopped flat-leaf parsley

In a bowl, soak the capers in 1 cup water for 10 minutes, then drain well.

In a large skillet, heat the oil over medium heat. Add the garlic and anchovy paste and cook until fragrant, 45 seconds to 1 minute. Stir in the tomatoes, capers, olives, oregano, and pepper flakes. After 2 to 3 minutes, begin crushing the tomatoes with the back of a spoon to create bite-size chunks of tomato. The longer the tomatoes cook, the more easily they will break up. Cook over medium-low heat until the sauce has developed a nice thick consistency, about 20 minutes.

In a medium pot of boiling water, cook the pasta according to package directions. Drain and serve topped with the sauce and a sprinkling of parsley to garnish.

Makes 4 servings
1 serving = 1 Reinforce carbohydrate &
1 vegetable carbohydrate & 1 fat

Juicy, Cheesy Spinach Turkey Burgers

The spinach and feta cheese add moisture to ground turkey breast, which has a tendency to be dry. Don't overcook the burgers. Omit the bun and this will be phase 2 friendly.

I pound ground turkey breast or extra-lean ground meat
½ cup crumbled reduced-fat feta cheese
½ cup chopped fresh spinach
½ teaspoon black pepper
½ teaspoon garlic salt or fresh garlic, minced
4 whole wheat burger buns
4 lettuce leaves (optional)
4 tomato slices (optional)

In a large bowl, combine the turkey, feta cheese, spinach, pepper, and garlic salt or garlic and blend gently but thoroughly. Form into 4 equal patties.

Grill the burgers or pan-fry in a hot nonstick skillet for about 6 minutes on 1 side. Turn and cook until no longer pink in the center, about 6 minutes.

Serve on a whole wheat bun. Add lettuce and tomato, if desired.

Makes 4 servings
I serving = I protein & I Reinforce carbohydrate &
I vegetable carbohydrate

Sides, Starters, and Snacks

PHASE I FRIENDLY

REIGNITE YOUR METABOLISM

WEEKS 1–2

French Green Beans with Garlic and Lemon

Make a triple batch of these flavorful green beans on the weekend when you have more time and use them as your veggie all during the week. They pair well with fish, chicken, or lean beef. If you like a little spice, add a pinch of red pepper flakes to give the beans a kick.

2 cups or about 9 ounces haricots verts (thin French green beans)
2 tablespoons fresh lemon juice
I teaspoon extra-virgin olive oil
I clove garlic, minced
Pinch of salt

Using your preferred method, steam the green beans until still bright green and just tender. You want them to have a mild crunch. Toss them with the lemon juice, oil, garlic, and salt.

Makes 1 or 2 servings
I serving = I vegetable carbohydrate

The Mile-High Protein Smoothie

This smoothie is perfect for breakfast or, if you're hungry for something sweet, as a dessert for your last meal of the day. Protein powder comes in a variety of flavors, giving you many options. For example, combine raspberry truffle protein powder with 1 tablespoon of sugar-free chocolate pudding mix for a dessert, or use banana extract and a banana or vanilla protein powder for a morning smoothie.

1 cup chilled fat-free milk or unsweetened almond milk
1 scoop protein powder (your favorite flavor)
Optional flavor-boosting add-ins: PB2, your favorite extract,
    or sugar-free syrup
About 1 cup ice cubes

Pour the milk or water into a blender, then add the protein powder (see Tip). Add a flavoring of your choice, if desired. Blend to a smooth consistency. Add ice cubes (1 cup or more, depending on how thick you want the smoothie) and blend for an additional 30 to 60 seconds on high speed.

Makes 1 serving
1 serving = 1 protein & 1 Reignite carbohydrate

Tip: *The order in which you add the ingredients to the blender matters. Always put the liquid in first to get the best blending.*

Roasted Eggplant with Garlic and Fresh Oregano

Pair this eggplant with grilled chicken breast or lean pork.

1 medium eggplant, about 1 pound, cut into 1" dice
2 tablespoons olive oil
Pinch of salt
Pinch of freshly ground black pepper
½ pint cherry tomatoes, halved
6 cloves garlic, finely chopped
3 tablespoons chopped fresh oregano
2 tablespoons red wine vinegar or balsamic vinegar

Preheat the oven to 350°F.

Toss the eggplant in the oil. Season with the salt and several turns of a pepper mill and toss again.

Place the eggplant in a roasting pan and roast until it starts to get tender (test with a fork), about 25 minutes. Add the tomatoes, garlic, and oregano and toss. Roast until the eggplant is tender and the vegetables are fragrant, another 10 to 15 minutes.

Transfer the roasted vegetables to a bowl and toss with the vinegar. Season to taste with salt and pepper.

Makes 4 servings
1 serving = 1 vegetable carbohydrate & 1 fat

Avocado Caprese Salad

A traditional caprese is made with fresh mozzarella, but it is difficult to find a good reduced-fat one, and avocados are a great, healthy substitute. The avocados deliver the creaminess you would get from the mozzarella, and the arugula gives the salad a little added nutty flavor to make it interesting. Combine this flavorful salad with some grilled lean bison for a special meal that is still phase 2 worthy.

6 ounces baby arugula
3 tomatoes, cut into ¼" slices
1 avocado, pitted, peeled, and sliced lengthwise into strips
2 handfuls of fresh basil leaves
2 tablespoons olive oil
3 teaspoons balsamic vinegar
Pinch of coarse salt
Pinch of coarsely ground black pepper

Layer the arugula on a platter. Arrange alternating slices of tomato, strips of avocado, and basil leaves on top. Drizzle the olive oil and vinegar over the top. Sprinkle with the salt and pepper.

Makes 2 or 3 servings
1 serving = 1 vegetable carbohydrate & 1 fat

PHASE 2
REBUILD YOUR METABOLISM
WEEKS 3–8

Brown and Wild Rice Medley

You can serve this rice with nearly any grilled or baked lean protein source, including fish, chicken, pork, or beef. If you want to give the rice an Asian flair, use toasted sesame oil instead of canola.

1 cup mixed brown and wild rice
1 cup low-sodium chicken broth
1 teaspoon canola oil
2 tablespoons finely chopped carrot
1 clove garlic, finely chopped
1 teaspoon minced fresh ginger
2 teaspoons reduced-sodium soy sauce
2 tablespoons minced flat-leaf parsley
2 tablespoons chopped scallion
¼ teaspoon freshly ground black pepper (or to taste)

In a saucepan, cook the rice mixture according to package directions in the broth and 1 cup water.

Meanwhile, in a separate nonstick saucepan, heat the oil over medium heat. Add the carrot, garlic, and ginger and cook until fragrant, about 3 minutes. Stir in the soy sauce and set aside.

When the rice is cooked, stir in the carrot mixture, parsley, and scallion. Add the pepper to taste. Serve hot.

Makes 4 servings
1 serving = 1 Rebuild carbohydrate

Creamy Butternut Squash Soup

The ground red pepper gives this soup subtle warmth. Some people like to add hot sauce to their bowl to kick "subtle" to a higher level. To make this a great phase 2 dinner, serve the soup with a lean pork chop or roasted chicken breast.

I butternut squash (2½–3 pounds), halved lengthwise and seeded
I tablespoon olive oil
½ cup diced onion
½ cup diced celery
½ cup diced carrot
8 cups low-sodium chicken broth
⅛ teaspoon ground red pepper
⅛ teaspoon freshly grated nutmeg (or more to taste)
½ cup low-fat or fat-free evaporated milk

Preheat the oven to 350°F. Line a baking sheet or roasting pan with foil.

Place the squash halves cut side down on the baking sheet and bake until the flesh is soft and tender, 35 to 45 minutes (depending on the size).

Meanwhile, in a Dutch oven or soup pot, heat the oil over medium heat. Add the onion, celery, and carrot and cook, stirring frequently, until softened, about 6 minutes.

In a large bowl, mix together the sautéed vegetables and the chicken broth. When the squash is soft, remove it from the oven and let it cool. Scoop the flesh out of the skin. Working in batches, puree the squash in a blender with some of the broth and vegetable mixture until smooth. Be careful blending the warm liquid, starting on low and gradually increasing the speed, and make sure your blender has a vent hole in the lid. As each batch is done, add the puree back to the pot and keep warm. Repeat this procedure until all the squash has been pureed.

Heat the soup over low to medium heat and stir in the ground red pepper and nutmeg. At this stage, you can adjust the thickness of the soup with the evaporated milk. If you started with a large squash, chances are you will have very thick soup and will want to add some milk to improve the consistency. Serve the soup when warmed all the way through.

Makes 10 servings
1 serving = 1 Rebuild carbohydrate

PHASE 2 FRIENDLY
_____
REBUILD YOUR METABOLISM
_____
WEEKS 3–8

Fiery Sweet Potato Chips

Add a lean grilled ground bison patty and you have a perfect Friday night dinner. You can make this same recipe with a regular baking potato in phase 3. If you do not like "fiery," omit the hot sauce.

2 tablespoons olive oil
1 tablespoon hot sauce
1 teaspoon ground cumin
1 teaspoon paprika
1 sweet potato (8–10 ounces), thinly sliced
Salt and freshly ground black pepper

Preheat the oven to 450°F. Lightly coat a baking sheet with cooking spray.

In a bowl, combine the oil, hot sauce, cumin, and paprika. Add the sweet potato slices and toss to coat.

Spread the sweet potato slices in a single layer on the baking sheet. Season to taste with a little salt and pepper. Bake for 12 to 15 minutes. Flip and bake until golden brown, about 15 minutes.

Makes 2 servings
1 serving = 1 Rebuild carbohydrate & 1 fat

PHASE 2 FRIENDLY

REBUILD YOUR METABOLISM

WEEKS 3–8

Fresh Basil, Garlic, and Lemon Hummus

This dish pairs well with herbed chicken or turkey as a protein accompaniment. Cut the cooked meat into small slices or chunks and serve on top of pita wedges with a smear of hummus.

Large handful of fresh basil leaves
1 clove garlic
1 tablespoon olive oil
1 tablespoon fresh lemon juice
1 can (15 ounces) chickpeas, drained, liquid reserved
Pinch of salt
Pinch of freshly ground black pepper
2 whole wheat pitas, cut into wedges

Preheat the oven to 300°F.

In a food processor, combine the basil, garlic, oil, and lemon juice and process until the basil is well chopped. Add the chickpeas and salt and pepper and blend until the mixture is smooth and free of lumps. Adjust the consistency with the liquid reserved from the can.

Spread the pita wedges on a baking sheet and bake until toasted, about 10 minutes.

Makes 4 servings
1 serving = 1 Rebuild carbohydrate

Vegetable Barley Soup with Chicken

You can add almost any vegetable to this soup to create variation. Try some leeks or baby bok choy. Look for vegetables that are in season. Add the green leafy vegetables at the very end, just before serving, so they retain their nice green color.

1 tablespoon olive oil
1 cup diced onion
1 cup diced carrot
1 cup diced celery
3 cloves garlic, finely chopped
3 quarts low-sodium chicken broth
1 cup pearled barley
3 pounds boneless, skinless chicken breasts cut into $\frac{1}{2}$" chunks
1 tablespoon dried oregano
2 tablespoons dried parsley
2 teaspoons dried basil
2 teaspoons dried thyme
1 bay leaf
$\frac{1}{4}$ teaspoon red pepper flakes
Pinch of salt
Pinch of freshly ground black pepper
1 zucchini, halved lengthwise and cut crosswise into $\frac{1}{4}$" half-moons
$\frac{1}{2}$ cup shelled edamame
$\frac{1}{2}$ cup frozen peas or sugar snap peas cut into thirds
3 ounces baby spinach or baby arugula

In a large soup pot, heat the oil over medium heat. Add the onion, carrot, celery, and garlic and cook until tender, about 8 minutes. Add the chicken broth and bring to a boil. Reduce the heat to medium and add the barley, chicken, oregano, parsley, basil, thyme, bay leaf, red pepper flakes, and salt and pepper. Simmer for 30 minutes.

Add the zucchini, edamame, and peas and simmer for 15 minutes. Add the spinach or arugula and stir until wilted. Adjust the seasoning to taste. Discard the bay leaf.

Makes 12 servings

I serving = I protein & I Rebuild carbohydrate &
I vegetable carbohydrate

Parmesan-Roasted Vegetables

If you are not a big fan of vegetables, you must try them roasted. It brings out the sweetness in the veggies and is the only way some people will eat them. Omit the cheese and you can serve this recipe in phases 1 and 2. Pair the roasted vegetables with a juicy rib eye and you have a fabulous, very satisfying dinner.

8 cups cauliflower florets (or Brussels sprouts, carrots, parsnips, beets, or turnips)
2 tablespoons olive oil
3–4 teaspoons freshly ground black pepper
Salt
3–4 tablespoons chopped fresh parsley
1 cup reduced-fat grated Parmesan cheese

Preheat the oven to 400°F. Lightly coat a baking sheet with olive oil spray.

In a large bowl, combine the cauliflower, oil, pepper, and salt to taste and toss to coat. Add the parsley and cheese and toss well to coat the vegetables with the oil and cheese.

Place the mixture on the pan and roast, uncovered and tossing once, until the vegetables are slightly browned and tender, 20 to 25 minutes. Serve warm.

Makes 4 servings
1 serving = 1 Reinforce carbohydrate &
1 vegetable carbohydrate & 1

PHASE 3 FRIENDLY
REINFORCE YOUR METABOLISM
WEEKS 9–16

"Sassy" Spinach with Sun-Dried Cherries and Roma Tomatoes

You can also make this dish with arugula instead of spinach. Add a phase 3 protein source and you will have a mile-high meal bursting with flavor.

2 teaspoons olive oil
3–4 cloves garlic, finely chopped
½ cup dried cherries, raisins, dried cranberries, or chopped dried apricots
2 Roma (plum) tomatoes, seeded and cut into ½" cubes
¼ teaspoon red pepper flakes (or more to taste)
I bag (9 ounces) prewashed spinach
⅛ teaspoon freshly grated nutmeg
Salt and freshly ground black pepper

In a large skillet, heat the oil over medium heat. Add the garlic and cook until softened, 1 to 2 minutes. Add the dried cherries or other fruit, tomatoes, and pepper flakes. Cook for another 1 to 2 minutes to soften the cherries and tomatoes.

Add the spinach and toss with tongs or 2 spoons until the spinach begins to wilt and reduce in volume. When the spinach is wilted, remove the pan from the heat. Season with the nutmeg and salt and pepper to taste. Toss with tongs or spoons to distribute the seasonings. Serve hot.

Makes 4 servings
I serving = I Reinforce carbohydrate &
I vegetable carbohydrate

Workout-Refueling Protein Shake

Drink this shake after a tough phase 3 workout: The protein and the simple sugar from the fruit are perfect after a workout—the sugar will help get the protein into your muscles. You can use any frozen fruit you like or make a chocolate variety using chocolate protein powder.

½ cup cold fat-free milk or unsweetened almond milk
½ cup water
1 scoop vanilla protein powder
½ small banana, frozen in 2" pieces
6 frozen strawberries
Ice cubes (as many as you like)

Pour the fat-free milk or almond milk and water into the blender, then add the protein powder (see Tip). Blend to a smooth consistency. Add the frozen banana and then the strawberries. Blend for 30 seconds. Add ice cubes if needed if you want a thinner shake. Blend for an additional 30 seconds to 1 minute on high speed. Pour into a tall glass.

Makes 1 serving
1 serving = 1 protein & 1 Reinforce carbohydrate

Tip: *The order in which you add the ingredients to the blender matters. Always put the liquid in first to get the best results.*

Spreads, Spices, and Sauces

PHASE I FRIENDLY

REIGNITE YOUR METABOLISM

WEEKS I–2

Greek Yogurt Cream Cheese

Yogurt cheese is very versatile. Try adding cinnamon, vanilla extract, and stevia for a sweet spread, or add garlic, salt, basil, and even spinach for a zesty high-protein dip or spread.

Nonfat plain Greek yogurt

Place 3 or 4 layers of cheesecloth in a fine-mesh sieve. Place the sieve over a large bowl. Add the Greek yogurt and let it drain for 12 hours in the refrigerator. The whey will drain out of the yogurt (and into the bowl), leaving soft cream cheese in the sieve. Store in an airtight container in the refrigerator.

8 ounces of Greek yogurt before straining = I protein

PHASE I FRIENDLY
REIGNITE YOUR METABOLISM
WEEKS I–2

Simple Homemade Pico de Gallo

While this is phase I friendly, it pairs well with many phase 2 and phase 3 dishes as well. You can customize your creation in lots of ways, such as by adding red bell pepper or mixing up the color with heirloom tomatoes.

3 large tomatoes, diced
I medium red onion, diced
I–2 fresh jalapeño chile peppers, seeded and chopped (keep the seeds if you like spice); wear plastic gloves when handling
I clove garlic, minced
3 tablespoons chopped cilantro
2 tablespoons fresh lemon juice
I teaspoon salt

In a medium bowl, stir together the tomatoes, onion, jalapeño peppers, garlic, cilantro, lemon juice, and salt. Cover and refrigerate for 30 minutes or longer to let the flavors blend. Store in a covered container in the refrigerator, where it will keep for at least 2 weeks.

Makes 3–4 cups
I cup = I vegetable carbohydrate

Lemon-Garlic Aioli

A great accompaniment to fish and chicken.

½ cup nonfat plain Greek yogurt
Juice of ½ lemon
1 large clove garlic, chopped or crushed through a press
⅛ teaspoon ground white pepper
Pinch of salt

In a small bowl, blend together the yogurt, lemon juice, garlic, white pepper, and salt. Cover and refrigerate for 30 minutes to 1 hour to let the flavors infuse before serving.

Makes about ½ cup
1 cup = 1 protein

Low-Salt Spice Mix/Rub

This rub is great for grilling lean pork, beef, and chicken. It also works well on white fish like halibut.

2 tablespoons plus 1½ teaspoons paprika

1 teaspoon salt

2 tablespoons garlic powder

1 tablespoon freshly ground black pepper

In a bowl, mix the paprika, salt, garlic powder, and pepper.

Makes about ⅓ cup
1 serving = a flavor booster

PHASE 2 FRIENDLY

REBUILD YOUR METABOLISM

WEEKS 3–8

Low-Fat Basil and Bean Pesto

This isn't a traditional pesto with pine nuts, cheese, and lots of olive oil, so this tastes different from regular pesto, but you will likely find that it has many uses for boosting the flavor of your dishes.

I cup packed fresh basil leaves
I clove garlic
I can (15 ounces) cannellini beans, drained, liquid reserved
3 tablespoons fresh lemon juice
I tablespoon olive oil
½ teaspoon fine sea salt

In a food processor, combine the basil, garlic, beans, lemon juice, oil, salt, and 1 tablespoon warm water. Process until smooth, adjusting the consistency with the liquid reserved from the can.

Makes about 2 cups
I cup = I Rebuild carbohydrate & I fat

Crunchy Mango Salsa

This salsa goes well with chicken or fish. When peaches are in season, you can use 2 medium-size ones in place of the mango. Peel, pit, and dice the peaches, as described for the mango.

1 mango, peeled, pitted, and diced (about 1½ cups)
½ medium red onion, finely chopped
½ small cucumber, peeled, seeded, and diced
¼ cup chopped red, yellow, or orange bell pepper
2 tablespoons chopped jicama (crunch enhancer; optional)
1 fresh jalapeño chile pepper, seeded and minced (wear plastic gloves when handling)
3 tablespoons chopped cilantro
3 tablespoons fresh lime juice
Salt and freshly ground black pepper
½ avocado, peeled and diced, for garnish (optional)

In a large bowl, toss together the mango, onion, cucumber, bell pepper, jicama (if using), jalapeño pepper, cilantro, and lime juice. Season to taste with salt and black pepper. Garnish the top of the salsa with a few chunks of the avocado, if using. (Don't mix it into the salsa, as it will get mushy.)

Makes about 3 cups
1.5 cups = 1 Reinforce carbohydrate &
1 vegetable carbohydrate

Resources

THIS SECTION PROVIDES LINKS to resources you might find helpful as you follow the Colorado Diet and live the Colorado lifestyle. Additional resources can be found on the official Colorado Diet Web site, stateofslim.com.

RESOURCES FOR HEALTHY EATING

- We like the following cookbooks for healthy recipes: (1) *The Food You Crave: Luscious Recipes for a Healthy Life,* by Ellie Krieger; (2) *Betty Crocker's Healthy New Choices: A Fresh Approach to Eating Well;* (3) *Betty Crocker Win at Weight Loss Cookbook: A Healthy Guide for the Whole Family* (with James O. Hill); (4) *American Heart Association Healthy Slow Cooker Cookbook;* and (5) *Tosca Reno's Eat Clean Cookbook,* by Tosca Reno.

- Healthy Dining Finder (healthydiningfinder.com) identifies restaurants that offer healthier choices.

- You don't need to count calories on the Colorado Diet, but it's useful to have a resource to identify the composition and energy content of specific foods. The CalorieKing book *(The CalorieKing Calorie, Fat, & Carbohydrate Counter)* and Web site (calorieking. com) provide this information for most foods.

- America On the Move is a nonprofit that encourages people to make small changes in diet and physical activity. Find their useful hints at americaonthemove.org. You need to join to get to the tips, but membership is free.

- Kitchen audit. See the Family Food Audit at https://aom3.america onthemove.org/Tools.aspx.

RESOURCES FOR PHYSICAL ACTIVITY

- For help in finding motivation for physical activity, we recommend the following books: *Motivating People to Be Physically Active,* 2nd ed., by Bess H. Marcus and LeighAnn Forsyth; and *Active Living Every Day with Online Resource,* 2nd ed., by Steven Blair, Andrea Dunn, Bess Marcus, Ruth Ann Carpenter, and Peter Jaret.

- *The Step Diet: Count Steps, Not Calories, to Lose Weight and Keep It Off Forever,* by James O. Hill, John C. Peters, and Bonnie Jortberg, offers great tips for becoming an active person.

- If you are looking for ideas on how and where to be active, try pbs. org/americaswalking/resources.html.

- Most communities have YMCAs. These provide a great place to start being active.

- Most towns and cities have parks and recreation departments that can direct you to places to be active at little or no cost. Check with your town's recreation department to see what's available.

- Most communities also have private gyms and fitness centers. You can get tips on how to find one that is right for you at the Web site of the International Health, Racquet & Sportsclub Association (IHRSA): healthclubs.com.

- America On the Move (americaonthemove.org) offers information on how to purchase and use a pedometer and how to start walking. You can also track your steps online.

- There are a large number of pedometers from manufacturers such as Omron, Yamax, Accusplit, New-Lifestyles, and others. Expect to pay $20 to $25 for a good pedometer. Several Web sites rate these devices, including walking.about.com/od/measure/tp/pedometer.htm. Novel forms of pedometers have looser placement requirements. For example, the Omron HJ-112 uses dual-axis accelerometers that detect not only vertical but also horizontal movements. This pedometer can be put in a pocket or bag, and it still takes step readings.

- Many devices measure total body movement and physical activity. Popular ones include the Fitbit (fitbit.com), Bodybugg (bodybugg.com), Nike FuelBand (nike.com/FuelBand), and Jawbone UP (jawbone.com/up).

- Looking to join a walking group or start your own? The Volkssport Association is a very popular walking club. Try the American Volkssport Association (ava.org) or its European counterpart, the International Federation of Popular Sports (ivv-web.org). The American Heart Association provides advice at startwalkingnow.org.

- A great way to meet people who enjoy physical activity is to sign up for a 5-K run or walk.

- To learn more about the benefits of resistance exercise and read tips for getting started, see mayoclinic.com/health/strength-training/HQ01710.

RESOURCES FOR ACQUIRING A COLORADO MIND-SET

- We like the book *Positivity,* by Barbara Fredrickson, to help you become an optimist.

- *The Power of Full Engagement,* by Jim Loehr and Tony Schwartz, explores the importance of identifying your purpose.

- Find in-depth information about sleep at http://healthfinder.gov/ Search/?q=sleep, where you can take an online quiz to assess your current sleep habits and get tips on improving.

- Build a personal mission statement. Visit franklincovey.com/msb.

- *The Path: Creating Your Mission Statement for Work and for Life,* by Laurie Beth Jones

- *Finding Your Own North Star: Claiming the Life You Were Meant to Live,* by Martha Beck

- *Soul Mission, Life Vision,* by Alan Seale

OTHER RESOURCES

- You can learn more about our research and our weight management programs at the Anschutz Health and Wellness Center at anschutzwellness.com.

- After you have lost at least 30 pounds and kept it off for a year, join the National Weight Control Registry online at nwcr.ws.

- Learn about our 5th Gear Kids wellness program for fifth graders at 5thgearkids.org.

Appendix I

SAMPLE DAILY MENUS

WHEN YOU CHANGE your diet, day-by-day, meal-by-meal eating plans can be both a blessing and a curse. On the one hand, it takes the guesswork out of what you should be eating—and that's especially helpful when you're just getting started and adapting to a new eating style. On the other, it can feel limiting (what if you don't want chicken for dinner on Tuesday or you don't like cauliflower?).

We firmly believe that you have to develop an eating strategy that works for *your* lifestyle and appeals to *your* taste buds, which is why we didn't include prescribed meal plans for each phase of the diet in the Colorado Diet phase chapters. However, we know that you might wonder what the Colorado Diet looks like in the real world—and you might need some guidance putting your protein, carb, and fat combos together. Here we've laid out a week's worth of meal suggestions for each phase of the plan. In addition to giving you some ideas, we think you'll be pleased to see just how varied and satisfying each phase of the Colorado Diet can be. Follow the sample days exactly, use them for inspiration, or both—it's totally up to you.

Phase 1: Reignite Your Metabolism

- Have a **protein** and a **carbohydrate** at every meal and snack.

- Three of your carb choices can be a **Reignite Carb.**

- **Vegetable Carbohydrates** should be your only carbohydrate choice for three meals each day. However, you can have as many and as much of them as you want; there are no limits on portion size for these foods. In addition, you can add unlimited amounts of Vegetable Carbohydrates to any meal.

- Have two **fat** servings a day.

Refer to the list on pages 120–121 for more choices in each category and remember to stick to the portion sizes given for the various foods.

DAY 1	PROTEIN	REIGNITE CARB	VEGETABLE CARB	FAT
Breakfast				
• Egg-White Omelet with Fresh Veggies (p. 181)	Egg whites	Fat-free milk or almond milk	Vegetables in omelet	
• Fat-free milk, almond milk, or café au lait (8 oz milk and 4 oz coffee)				
Snack				
• Nonfat Greek yogurt seasoned to taste with garlic powder and dried herbs, such as basil, oregano, rosemary, and parsley	Greek yogurt		Assorted vegetables	
• Assorted sliced vegetables				
Lunch				
• Chicken gazpacho salad: *Toss mixed salad greens, cherry tomatoes, cucumber, scallions, celery, and finely minced garlic with red wine vinegar and 1 Tbsp olive oil. Top with sliced cooked chicken.*	Chicken		Salad greens Vegetables in salad	Olive oil
Snack				
• Oatmeal	Cottage cheese	Oatmeal		
• Fat-free cottage cheese				
Dinner				
• Baked Salmon with Mustard Dill Sauce (p. 186)	Salmon		Green beans	Salmon
• French Green Beans with Garlic and Lemon (p. 207)				
Snack				
The Mile-High Protein Smoothie (p. 208)	Protein powder	Fat-free milk or almond milk		

DAY 2	PROTEIN	REIGNITE CARB	VEGETABLE CARB	FAT
Breakfast				
• Cinnamon-Pumpkin Protein Pancakes (p. 180)	Protein powder Egg whites	Pumpkin Oats		
Snack				
• Fat-free cottage cheese mixed with lemon zest and freshly ground black pepper, with baby carrots and snow peas	Cottage cheese	Fat-free milk or almond milk	Carrots Snow peas	
• Fat-free milk, almond milk, or café au lait (8 oz milk and 4 oz coffee)				
Lunch				
• Herbed Chicken Roll-Ups with Spinach and Roasted Red Pepper (p. 190)	Chicken		Spinach Roasted red pepper	
Snack				
• Steamed asparagus tossed with chopped egg whites, chopped fresh chives, and 1 Tbsp olive oil	Egg whites		Asparagus	Olive oil
Dinner				
• Grilled sirloin steak	Sirloin		Cauliflower	
• Roasted balsamic cauliflower: *Toss cauliflower florets with salt, pepper, and 1 tsp olive oil. Spread on a foil-lined baking sheet and roast in a 450°F oven for 15 to 20 minutes until the cauliflower begins to get tender. Remove from oven, drizzle with balsamic vinegar, and continue roasting for 10 to 15 minutes.*				
Snack				
• Chocolate Cheesecake Muffins (p. 178)	Protein powder	Oats		Walnuts
• Toasted walnuts				

DAY 3	PROTEIN	REIGNITE CARB	VEGETABLE CARB	FAT
Breakfast				
• Protein-packed oatmeal: *Stir 1 scoop chocolate or vanilla protein powder into cooked oatmeal.*	Protein powder	Oats		
Snack				
• Nonfat Greek yogurt with sugar-free jam or syrup	Greek yogurt	Fat-free milk or almond milk		Almonds
• Fat-free milk, almond milk, or café au lait (8 oz milk and 4 oz coffee)				
• Roasted almonds				
Lunch				
• Beef burger (made with very lean ground beef) seasoned with Low-Salt Spice Mix (p. 224)	Beef		Pico de Gallo	Olive oil
• Simple Homemade Pico de Gallo (p. 222)			Salad greens	
• Garden salad: *Toss mixed greens and assorted vegetables with an olive oil–based dressing.*			Vegetables in salad	
Snack				
• Endive leaves with Greek Yogurt Cream Cheese (p. 221): *Mix yogurt cheese with garlic powder and chopped pimiento peppers. Spoon into raw endive leaves.*	Greek yogurt		Endive Pimiento peppers	
Dinner				
• Crowd-Pleasing Slow-Cooker Pumpkin Chili (p. 194)	Ground beef or turkey	Pumpkin		
Snack				
• Chicken lettuce rolls: *Stir chopped cooked chicken breast into Simple Homemade Pico de Gallo (p. 222). Spread mixture on Romaine lettuce leaves and roll up.*	Chicken		Romaine lettuce Pico de Gallo	

DAY 4	PROTEIN	REIGNITE CARB	VEGETABLE CARB	FAT
Breakfast				
• Chocolate Cheesecake Muffins (p. 178)	Greek yogurt	Oats		
	Egg whites			
	Protein powder			
Snack				
• Fat-free cottage cheese mixed with cinnamon	Cottage cheese	Fat-free milk or almond milk		
• Fat-free milk, almond milk, or café au lait (8 oz milk and 4 oz coffee)				
Lunch				
• Chicken-walnut salad on endive: *Mix 6 oz. diced cooked chicken breast with 2 Tbsp nonfat mayo or yogurt, diced celery, onion, diced red peppers. Add 9 chopped walnut halves.*	Chicken		Endive Celery Onion Red peppers	Walnuts
Snack				
• Nonfat Greek yogurt seasoned to taste with garlic powder and dried herbs, such as basil, oregano, rosemary, and parsley	Greek yogurt		Assorted vegetables	
• Assorted sliced vegetables				
Dinner				
• Chicken and veggie "pasta": *Using a vegetable peeler, peel long thin strips of carrot, zucchini, and asparagus. Blanch briefly in salted boiling water. Toss with 4 oz cooked chicken and ½ cup marinara sauce.*	Chicken		Vegetables Marinara sauce	
Snack				
• The Mile-High Protein Smoothie (p. 208)	Protein powder	Fat-free milk or almond milk		Almonds
• Almonds				

DAY 5	PROTEIN	REIGNITE CARB	VEGETABLE CARB	FAT
Breakfast				
• Egg-White Omelet with Fresh Veggies (p. 181) • Fat-free milk, almond milk, or café au lait (8 oz milk and 4 oz coffee)	Egg whites	Fat-free milk or almond milk	Vegetables in omelet	
Snack				
• Chocolate Cheesecake Muffins (p. 178)	Greek yogurt Egg whites Protein powder	Oats		
Lunch				
• Crowd-Pleasing Slow-Cooker Pumpkin Chili (p. 194) • Garden salad: *Toss mixed greens and assorted vegetables with an olive oil–based dressing.*	Ground beef or turkey	Pumpkin	Salad greens Vegetables in chili and salad	Olive oil
Snack				
• Fat-free cottage cheese mixed with lemon zest and freshly ground black pepper with baby carrots and snow peas	Cottage cheese		Baby carrots Snow peas	
Dinner				
• Southwestern Chicken with Cilantro Cream Dipping Sauce (p. 192) • Roasted Eggplant with Garlic and Fresh Oregano (p. 209)	Chicken		Eggplant Tomatoes	Olive oil
Snack				
• Nonfat Greek yogurt with sugar-free jam or syrup • Walnuts	Greek yogurt			Walnuts

DAY 6	PROTEIN	REIGNITE CARB	VEGETABLE CARB	FAT
Breakfast				
• The Mile-High Protein Smoothie (p. 208)	Protein powder	Fat-free milk or almond milk		
Snack				
• Nonfat Greek yogurt seasoned to taste with garlic powder and dried herbs, such as basil, oregano, rosemary, and parsley	Greek yogurt		Assorted vegetables	
• Assorted sliced vegetables				
Lunch				
• Herb tuna salad: *Combine mixed greens with either fresh flat-leaf parsley, watercress, or fresh basil. Add cherry tomatoes, scallions, green beans, and radishes. Add 6 oz of drained water-packed tuna. Whisk 1 Tbsp olive oil, Dijon mustard, and white vinegar for a dressing.*	Tuna		Salad greens Vegetables in salad	Olive oil
Snack				
• Endive leaves with Greek Yogurt Cream Cheese (p. 221): *Mix yogurt cheese with garlic powder and chopped pimiento peppers. Spoon into raw endive leaves.*	Greek yogurt		Endive leaves Pimiento peppers	
Dinner				
• Roasted or grilled turkey cutlet or chicken breast	Turkey or chicken	Pumpkin	Green beans	
• Pumpkin with sage: *Sauté chopped red onion or shallots in a nonstick skillet sprayed with cooking spray until soft. Add canned pumpkin and stir to heat through. Season with salt, freshly ground black pepper, and chopped fresh sage.*				
• French Green Beans with Garlic and Lemon (p. 207)				
Snack				
• Protein-packed oatmeal: *Stir 1 scoop chocolate or vanilla protein powder into cooked oatmeal.*	Protein powder	Oats		Almonds
• Toasted almonds				

DAY 7 Breakfast	PROTEIN	REIGNITE CARB	VEGETABLE CARB	FAT
• Egg white salad stacks: *Combine chopped egg whites with chopped red onion, chopped celery, chopped red peppers, lemon juice, Dijon mustard, and nonfat mayo. Serve on 4 thick slices of large beefsteak tomatoes.* • Fat-free milk, almond milk, or café au lait (8 oz milk and 4 oz coffee)	Egg whites	Fat-free milk or almond milk	Vegetables in egg salad Tomatoes	
Snack				
• Fat-free cottage cheese mixed with lemon zest and freshly ground black pepper with baby carrots and snow peas	Cottage cheese		Carrots Snow peas	
Lunch				
• Steak salad: *Sliced sirloin on a bed of greens with red peppers, tomatoes, onion, and green beans drizzled with a red wine vinegar/olive oil dressing.*	Steak		Salad greens Vegetables in salad	Olive oil
Snack				
• Pumpkin pie yogurt: *Mix 8 oz nonfat Greek yogurt with ¼ cup canned pumpkin, cinnamon, and pumpkin pie spice.*	Greek yogurt	Pumpkin		
Dinner				
• Chicken Tenders with Spicy Summer Squash (p. 188) • Garden salad: *Toss mixed greens and assorted vegetables with an olive oil–based dressing.*	Chicken		Summer squash Vegetables in salad	Olive oil
Snack				
• The Mile-High Protein Smoothie (p. 208)	Protein powder	Fat-free milk or almond milk		

Phase 2: Rebuild Your Metabolism

- Have a **protein** and a **carbohydrate** at every meal and snack.

- Three of your carbs each day can be a **Rebuild Carb.** Only two of those choices should be a carb added in this phase. These new carbs are highlighted in bold.

- **Vegetable Carbohydrates** should be your only carbohydrate choice for the other 3 meals. However, you can have as many and as much of them as you want; there are no limits on portion size for these foods. In addition, you can add unlimited amounts of Vegetable Carbs to any meal.

- Have two **fat** servings a day.

Refer to the list on pages 142–144 for more choices in each category and remember to stick to the portion sizes given for the various foods. **Boldface** references foods added in this phase.

DAY 1	PROTEIN	REBUILD CARB	VEGETABLE CARB	FAT
Breakfast				
• Protein-packed oatmeal: *Stir 1 scoop chocolate or vanilla protein powder into cooked oatmeal.*	Protein powder	Oatmeal		Pistachios
• Pistachios				
Snack				
• Tuna mixed with 1 chopped cucumber, 1 tsp olive oil, freshly ground black pepper, and chopped dill	Tuna		Cucumber	
Lunch				
• Herb Chicken Roll-Ups with Spinach and Roasted Red Peppers (p. 190)	Chicken	**Ezekiel bread**	Spinach Roasted red peppers	
• Ezekiel bread				
Snack				
• Greek Yogurt Cream Cheese (p. 221) mixed with garlic powder, freshly ground black pepper, and finely chopped spinach	Greek yogurt		Spinach in dip Assorted vegetables	
• Assorted sliced vegetables				
Dinner				
• Avocado Caprese Salad (p. 210)	Beef or buffalo		Arugula Tomatoes	Avocado
• Grilled beef or buffalo steak rubbed with herbs and 1 tsp olive oil				
Snack				
• Apple pie yogurt: *Mix nonfat Greek yogurt with chopped apple and cinnamon.*	Greek yogurt	**Apple**		

DAY 2	PROTEIN	REBUILD CARB	VEGETABLE CARB	FAT
Breakfast				
• Egg White Omelet with Fresh Veggies (p. 181) made with one egg and three egg whites • ½ grapefruit	Egg and egg whites	**Grapefruit**	Vegetables in omelet	
Snack				
• Chicken-guac pita: *Puree ⅓ avocado with red onion, cilantro, and lime juice. Mix in chopped tomatoes. Stuff a whole wheat pita with sliced cooked chicken and top with guacamole.*	Chicken	**Whole wheat pita**		**Avocado**
Lunch				
• Mediterranean tuna salad: *Mixed greens, sliced bell peppers, chopped red onion, olives, tuna, and lemon juice or balsamic vinegar*	Tuna		Salad greens Bell peppers Onion	Olives
Snack				
• Greek Yogurt Cream Cheese (p. 221) mixed with garlic powder, freshly ground black pepper, and finely chopped spinach • Assorted sliced vegetables	Greek yogurt		Spinach in dip Assorted vegetables	
Dinner				
• Beef-lettuce tacos: *Mix cooked ground beef with Simple Homemade Pico de Gallo (p. 222) diced tomatoes, diced green peppers, and 1 Tbsp taco seasoning mix. Wrap beef in leaves of Romaine lettuce.*	Ground beef		Pico de Gallo Tomatoes Green peppers Romaine lettuce	
Snack				
• The Mile-High Protein Smoothie (p. 208) made with 1 scoop chocolate protein powder and 2 Tbsp PB2	Protein powder	Fat-free milk or almond milk		

DAY 3	PROTEIN	REBUILD CARB	VEGETABLE CARB	FAT
Breakfast				
• Poached egg with asparagus: *One egg sprinkled with chili powder, sea salt, and freshly ground black pepper. Serve with sautéed asparagus and onions.*	Egg		Asparagus Onions	
Snack				
• Nonfat Greek yogurt with berries	Greek yogurt	**Berries**		
Lunch				
• Savory Pork Taco Salad with Wilted Arugula (p. 196) served with extra greens instead of the tortilla	Pork		Arugula Pico de gallo	Avocado
• Simple Homemade Pico de Gallo (p. 222)				
• Sliced avocado				
Snack				
• Egg salad pita: *Chop 3 hard-boiled egg whites. Combine with diced celery and onion, fat-free mayo, and dried oregano. Stuff in 1 whole wheat pita.*	Egg whites	**Whole wheat pita**	Celery Onion	
Dinner				
• Chicken and roasted tomatoes: *Chicken breast rubbed with Low Salt Spice Mix/Rub (p. 224) topped with roasted cherry tomatoes drizzled with 1 tsp olive oil*	Chicken		Tomatoes Vegetable soup	
• Vegetable soup				
Snack				
• Chocolate Cheesecake Muffins (p. 178)	Greek yogurt	Oats		Walnuts
• Toasted walnuts	Egg whites Protein powder			

DAY 4	PROTEIN	REBUILD CARB	VEGETABLE CARB	FAT
Breakfast				
• Chocolate Cheesecake Muffins (p. 178)	Greek yogurt	Oats		
	Egg whites			
	Protein powder			
Snack				
• Greek Yogurt Cream Cheese (p. 221) mixed with 2 tbsp PB2	Greek yogurt	**Ezekiel bread**		
• 1 slice Ezekiel bread				
Lunch				
• Southwestern Chicken with Cilantro Cream Dipping Sauce (p. 192)	Chicken		Broccoli	
• Steamed broccoli drizzled with balsamic vinegar				
Snack				
• Fat-free cottage cheese with lemon juice, garlic powder, sea salt, and freshly ground black pepper	Cottage cheese		Assorted vegetables	
• Assorted vegetables				
Dinner				
• Baked Salmon with Mustard-Dill Sauce (p. 186)	Salmon		Zucchini	Salmon
• Steamed baby zucchini tossed with 1 tsp olive oil and ½ cup chopped fresh flat-leaf parsley			Parsley	
Snack				
• Nonfat Greek yogurt with berries	Greek yogurt	**Berries**		Walnuts
• Toasted walnuts				

DAY 5	PROTEIN	REBUILD CARB	VEGETABLE CARB	FAT
Breakfast				
• Cinnamon-Pumpkin Protein Pancakes (p. 180)	Protein powder	Pumpkin		Almonds
• Toasted almonds				
Snack				
• Endive leaves with Greek Yogurt Cream Cheese (p. 221): *Mix yogurt cheese with garlic powder and chopped pimento peppers. Spoon into raw endive leaves.*	Greek yogurt		Endive	
Lunch				
• Chicken salad: *Mixed greens, fresh basil, cherry tomatoes, chopped assorted vegetables, and roast chicken with an olive oil-based dressing*	Chicken	**Apple**	Salad greens Cherry tomatoes Assorted vegetables	Olive oil
• Apple				
Snack				
• 6 oz Canadian bacon, sliced, mixed with fresh spinach, grated carrots, and 1 Tbsp balsamic vinegar	Canadian bacon		Carrots Spinach	
Dinner				
• Indulgence meal				
Snack				
• Protein-packed oatmeal: *Stir 1 scoop chocolate or vanilla protein powder into cooked oatmeal.*	Protein powder	Oats		

DAY 6	PROTEIN	REBUILD CARB	VEGETABLE CARB	FAT
Breakfast				
• Egg White Omelet with Fresh Veggies (p. 181) • Fat-free milk, almond milk, or café au lait (8 oz milk and 4 oz coffee)	Egg whites	Fat-free milk or almond milk	Vegetables in omelet	
Snack				
• Nonfat cottage cheese mixed with herbs • Snow peas • Cauliflower florets • Almonds	Cottage cheese		Snow peas Cauliflower	Almonds
Lunch				
• Fabulous Fish Tacos (p. 198) • Mixed green salad with assorted vegetables	Fish	**Whole wheat tortilla**	Cabbage in tacos Salad greens Assorted vegetables	
Snack				
• Tomato soup • Hard-boiled egg	Egg		Tomato soup	
Dinner				
• Spice-Rubbed Pork Tenderloin with Balsamic Reduction (p. 202) • Steamed baby zucchini tossed with olive oil and ½ cup chopped fresh flat-leaf parsley • Mixed green salad with olive oil dressing	Pork		Zucchini Parsley Salad greens	Olive oil
Snack				
• Greek Yogurt Cream Cheese (p. 221) mixed with 2 tbsp PB2 • 1 slice Ezekiel bread	Greek yogurt	**Ezekiel bread**		

DAY 7	PROTEIN	REBUILD CARB	VEGETABLE CARB	FAT
Breakfast				
• Greek yogurt and mixed berries	Greek yogurt	**Berries**		
Snack				
• Fat-free milk, almond milk, or café au lait (8 oz milk and 4 oz coffee)	Canadian bacon	Fat-free milk or almond milk	Asparagus	
• Asparagus-bacon wraps: *Wrap roasted or steamed asparagus spears with Canadian bacon. Drizzle with 1 Tbsp balsamic vinegar.*				
Lunch				
• Beef burger (no bun)	Burger		Onion	Olive oil
• Onion and tomato salad with olive oil dressing			Tomato	
Snack				
• Nonfat cottage cheese mixed with lemon zest and freshly ground black pepper	Cottage cheese		Carrots	
• Baby carrots and snow peas			Snow peas	
Dinner				
• Grilled chicken or turkey breast	Chicken or turkey		Green beans	
• French Green Beans with Garlic and Lemon (p. 207)				
Snack				
• Chocolate Cheesecake Muffins (p. 178)	Protein powder	Oats		Almonds
• Almonds				

Phase 3: Reinforce Your Metabolism

- Have a **protein** and a **carbohydrate** at every meal and snack.
- Three of your carbs each day can be a **Reinforce Carb.** Unlike in phase 2, you can pick any option on the Reinforce Carb list (including new options highlighted in bold) for all 3 meals.
- **Vegetable Carbohydrates** should be your only carbohydrate choice for the other 3 meals. However, you can have as many and as much of them as you want; there are no limits on portion size for these foods. In addition, you can add unlimited amounts of Vegetable Carbs to any meal.
- Have two **fat** servings a day. (Oil is used in some of the recipes. If it accounts for 1 tsp or less of oil per serving, it does not count toward your daily fat servings.)

Refer to the list on pages 156–159 for more choices in each category and remember to stick to the portion sizes given for the various foods. **Boldface** references foods added in this phase.

DAY 1	PROTEIN	REINFORCE CARB	VEGETABLE CARB	FAT
Breakfast				
• Sausage and Egg Mile-High Muffin (p. 185)	Sausage Egg	**Whole grain muffin** **Reduced-fat cheese**		
Snack				
• Ham and carrot rolls with Lemon-Garlic Aioli (p. 223): *Roll carrot sticks in ham and drizzle with aioli.*	Ham		Carrots	Almonds
• Almonds				
Lunch				
• Juicy Cheesy Spinach Turkey Burger (p. 206)	Turkey	**Low-fat feta** **Whole wheat bun**		
Snack				
• Artichoke with cottage cheese dip: *Mix fat-free cottage cheese with herbs. Serve as a dip with steamed artichoke.*	Cottage cheese		Artichoke	
Dinner				
• Creamy Butternut Squash Soup (p. 212)	Shrimp	Wild rice	Butternut squash soup	Olive oil
• Pan Sautéed Shrimp with Wild Rice Medley (p. 201)				
Snack				
• Protein bar	Protein bar		Vegetables	
• Sliced raw vegetables				

DAY 2	PROTEIN	REINFORCE CARB	VEGETABLE CARB	FAT
Breakfast				
• Protein-packed oatmeal: Stir I scoop chocolate or vanilla protein powder into cooked oatmeal.	Protein powder	Oatmeal		Almonds
• Toasted almonds				
Snack				
• Lemon-Chia Seed Muffins (p. 183)	Protein powder	Oats **Nonfat lemon yogurt**		
Lunch				
• Indulgence meal				
Snack				
• Nonfat Greek yogurt with fresh blueberries	Greek yogurt	Blueberries		
Dinner				
• Spice-Rubbed Pork Tenderloin with Balsamic Reduction (p. 202) • Grilled zucchini and summer squash tossed with fresh parsley and olive oil	Pork		Zucchini Summer squash	Olive oil
Snack				
• Cilantro Cream Dipping Sauce (p. 193), I cup, with broccoli and cauliflower florets	Greek yogurt in dip		Broccoli Cauliflower	

DAY 3	PROTEIN	REINFORCE CARB	VEGETABLE CARB	FAT
Breakfast				
• Sausage-veggie omelet: *Made with 1 egg and 2 egg whites, chopped onion, chopped red and green peppers, sliced mushrooms, and spinach. Crumble 1 lean turkey sausage patty into the egg and vegetable mixture, or serve it on the side.*	Sausage Egg		Vegetables in omelet	
Snack				
• Workout-Refueling Protein Shake (p. 220)	Protein powder	Fat-free milk or almond milk **Banana** Strawberries		
Lunch				
• Vegetable Barley Soup with Chicken (p. 216) • Garden salad: *Toss mixed greens and assorted vegetables with an olive-oil based dressing.*	Chicken	Barley	Assorted vegetables in soup and salad Salad greens	Olive oil
Snack				
• Whole grain bagel thin with peanut butter • Nonfat fruit Greek yogurt	Nonfat Greek yogurt	**Bagel thin**		Peanut butter
Dinner				
• Grilled New York strip steak • "Sassy" Spinach with Sun-Dried Cherries and Roma Tomatoes (p. 219)	Steak		Spinach Tomatoes	
Snack				
• Hard-boiled egg • Assorted sliced vegetables	Egg		Assorted vegetables	

DAY 4	PROTEIN	REINFORCE CARB	VEGETABLE CARB	FAT
Breakfast				
• Yogurt parfait: *Mix Kashi Go Lean Crunch cereal into blueberry nonfat Greek yogurt.*	Greek yogurt	**Kashi Go Lean Crunch cereal**		
Snack				
• Lemon–Chia Seed Muffin (p. 183)	Protein powder in muffin	Oats in muffin Lemon yogurt in muffin		
Lunch				
• Club sandwich: *Spread 2 slices reduced-calorie whole grain bread with 2 Tbsp nonfat mayo mixed with 1 tsp mustard. Top with lean ham, lean turkey, and 2 slices turkey bacon, cucumber, tomato, red onion, and lettuce.* • Pistachios	Ham Turkey Turkey bacon	**Reduced-calorie whole grain bread**		Pistachios
Snack				
• Creamy Butternut Squash Soup (p. 212) • Hard-boiled egg	Egg		Butternut squash soup	
Dinner				
• Pan-Seared Salmon with Chili Oil (p. 199) served on a bed of greens instead of wild rice • Roasted carrots	Salmon		Salad greens Carrots	Salmon
Snack				
• Protein bar • Assorted sliced vegetables	Protein bar		Assorted vegetables	

DAY 5	PROTEIN	REINFORCE CARB	VEGETABLE CARB	FAT
Breakfast				
• Very Berry Energizing Oatmeal (p. 182)	Protein powder	Oats Berries		
Snack				
• Fresh Basil, Garlic, and Lemon Hummus (p. 215) • Sliced red peppers and carrots • Deli ham	Ham	Pitas Chickpeas	Red peppers Carrots	
Lunch				
• Chicken salad with egg: *Top spinach and arugula with sliced chicken, I hard-boiled egg, celery, cherry tomatoes, and toasted slivered almonds.*	Chicken Egg		Spinach Arugula Vegetables in salad	Almonds
Snack				
• Protein bar • Snow peas	Protein bar		Snow peas	
Dinner				
• Indulgence meal				
Snack				
• Flavored nonfat Greek yogurt • Ezekiel bread • I Tbsp peanut butter or almond butter	Greek yogurt	Ezekiel bread		Peanut butter or almond butter

DAY 6	PROTEIN	REINFORCE CARB	VEGETABLE CARB	FAT
Breakfast				
• Sausage and Egg Mile-High Muffin (p. 185) made with Canadian bacon or sausage	Egg Sausage or Canadian bacon	**Muffin** **Cheese**		
Snack				
• Lemon–Chia Seed Muffin (p. 183)	Protein powder in muffin	Oats in muffin Lemon yogurt in muffin		
Lunch				
• Shrimp salad roll-up: *Mix nonfat mayo, 1 tsp mustard, ½ tsp Old Bay seasoning and diced celery and onion. Place on Boston or Bibb lettuce leaves. Top with shrimp and roll.* • Fennel and almond salad: *With a vegetable peeler, shave strips of fennel. Toss with toasted chopped almonds, lemon juice, and salt and freshly ground black pepper.*	Shrimp		Lettuce Fennel	Almonds
Snack				
• String cheese • Deli roast beef • Carrots and cherry tomatoes	Roast beef	String cheese	Cherry tomatoes Carrots	
Dinner				
• Roast chicken or turkey • Parmesan-Roasted Vegetables (p. 218) • Mixed greens with olive oil–based dressing	Chicken or turkey		Greens Vegetables	Olive oil
Snack				
• Nonfat Greek yogurt with sugar-free jam or syrup • Baby carrots	Greek yogurt		Baby carrots	

DAY 7	PROTEIN	REINFORCE CARB	VEGETABLE CARB	FAT
Breakfast				
• Protein bar	Protein bar		Baby carrots	
• Baby carrots				
Snack				
• Egg salad stacks: *Combine 1 chopped hard-boiled egg with chopped red onion, chopped celery, chopped red pepper, lemon juice, Dijon mustard, and nonfat mayo. Serve on 4 thick slices of large beefsteak tomatoes.*	Egg		Tomatoes Vegetables in egg salad	
Lunch				
• Low-Fat Basil and Bean Pesto (p. 225) with whole wheat pasta and chicken	Chicken	Beans in pesto **Whole wheat pasta**		
Snack				
• Goat cheese, arugula, and beet salad with an olive oil–based dressing	Turkey	**Goat cheese**		Olive oil
• Deli turkey				
Dinner				
• Ribeye steak	Steak	**Potato**	Cauliflower Broccoli	Walnuts
• Baked potato topped with a dollop of nonfat Greek yogurt and chopped chives				
• Roasted broccoli and cauliflower with toasted walnuts				
Snack				
• Nonfat Greek yogurt with sugar-free jam or syrup	Greek yogurt		Carrots	
• Baby carrots				

Appendix II

HEALTHY HABITS, ROUTINES, RITUALS, AND TIPS

THE MORE YOU ARE able to make healthy choices automatic, the easier it will be to remain in the state of slim. Here are some ideas. See which ones work for you.

HEALTHY EATING HABITS, ROUTINES, RITUALS, AND TIPS

- **The 15-minute hunger routine:** Whenever you are hungry other than at mealtime, ask yourself, "Am I really hungry?" Don't eat anything for at least 15 minutes and see if your body is telling you it is truly hungry or whether the feeling passes. You'll be surprised at how often the feeling disappears. If the hunger persists, use one of your six daily Colorado Diet meals to put the feeling to rest.

- **The six-meals-per-day routine:** Eat six meals every day. Have a specific plan for what you'll eat and when and where you'll eat it.

Have everything you need on hand so you're not tempted by impulse purchases during the day.

- **The breakfast routine:** Try eating the same breakfast every day during the workweek. Breakfast tends to be the least variable meal for most people, and eating the same food provides great structure for everyday success. You can mix it up on weekends.

- **Eat to savor:** Pretend every bite of food is the last bite you'll ever eat. Savor it in every dimension. Above all, slow down when you eat! Eating faster is associated with eating more.

- **The "8 x 8" routine:** Drink at least eight 8-ounce glasses of water each day. Drink a glass first thing in the morning, have one with each of your six meals, and have another after your last meal. This will ensure that you're well hydrated and keep hunger at bay.

- **The "take your lunch" routine:** Try taking your lunch every day of the week (if you work outside the home). You're almost guaranteed to eat more healthfully when you pack your own rather than try to navigate the nutritional landmine–laden world of fast-food and casual-dining restaurants.

- **Develop a weekly lunch menu** (for example, a certain menu for Mondays, Tuesdays, Wednesdays, etc.) to provide more structure to your meal plan and make food shopping easier. If you eat the same thing a few days a week, you'll know which ingredients always to have on hand to make lunch.

- **Downsize your plates:** Use smaller dishes for your meals at home. If you don't own smaller plates and bowls, you can purchase them in inexpensive sets. Many studies have shown that using smaller plates reduces how much food is eaten. Put your larger plates in a closet out of sight or donate them to a charity.

- **The preportioned snack routine:** Whenever you prepare a snack, always take a sensible portion and place it on a plate or bowl before you eat. You don't want to open a big bag of something and sit down to a bottomless snack!

- **The "be thankful" mealtime ritual:** Before eating, take a moment to count your blessings and be grateful for what you have. Think about where your food came from and give thanks for the bounty of nature.

- **The "doggie bag first" routine:** When you dine out, ask for a doggie bag container when you order and request that the waiter bring it when the food is served. Take half the food on your plate and put it in the container *before* you start eating. This saves you from the portion distortion that is prevalent in most restaurants. If you feel uncomfortable doing this up front, divide each item on your plate in half and put it on a separate plate to "keep it out of play." Then put it in the doggie bag at the end of the meal.

- **The "dressing/sauce on the side" habit:** In restaurants, ask for any dressing or sauce to be served on the side. These are usually high in fat and sodium, and you can use much less on your food than what is provided without sacrificing taste.

- **The "noncaloric beverage" routine:** Drink noncaloric beverages for most of your fluid intake. Once you reach the end phases of the Colorado Diet and are allowed the occasional small glass of fruit juice, choose the *one* you will build into your routine—for example, one 6-ounce serving of OJ in the morning. Beverages with calories do not provide much satiety and are typically the source of extra calories that will derail your healthy eating plan.

- **The "don't eat after 8:00 p.m." routine:** Don't eat anything after 8:00 in the evening. This gives your body a chance to process and integrate your food intake and activity for the day so your metabolism is ready to go first thing the next morning. You may wake up less hungry when you develop this routine.

- **Repackage bulk items:** Many foods come in bulk packs these days. If you aren't careful, you might dig in and eat more than one serving at a time. When you get home from the store, repack bulk items as single servings in zipper-lock bags or reusable containers. This portion control reduces the temptation to overdo it.

- **Get a kitchen scale** and weigh what you eat to learn what's an appropriate portion size. You'll be surprised at how fast you master portions, and then you won't need the scale as often.

- **Start a healthy cooking club** with local friends or family. Organize healthy progressive dinners once a month with your group or in your neighborhood.

PHYSICAL ACTIVITY ROUTINES, RITUALS, AND TIPS

- **Get specific:** Don't leave your daily activity to chance or wait till the last minute. Specify what activity you'll do each day and when and where you'll do it. Put it on your to-do list and have your gear ready.

- **Commit, don't quit:** Once you've scheduled your daily activity, don't schedule other things or bail out because "something came up." Let the people you work or live with know your intentions; this way, when you need to stay on schedule, they won't be offended if you leave to keep your workout appointment.

- **The "eat, then move your feet" routine:** Take a walk every day after lunch. It doesn't have to be a long excursion. You'd be surprised at how much energy you gain for the afternoon by taking a 10- to 15-minute walk after your meal.

- **The "weekend activity" ritual:** Plan a fun activity for every Saturday and Sunday. Involve family and friends, if possible. It can be anything lively and enjoyable. Go to the zoo or the museum or the park. Or walk the local shopping mall. When the weather's nice, head out for a bike ride or a long hike with a picnic lunch.

- **The more, the merrier:** Plan your activities with friends whenever possible. The support you give each other will be terrific, and it's harder to bail out if others are involved. Besides, talking while you work out make the time go faster.

- **The "don't sit still" routine:** Avoid sitting for prolonged periods. At work, stand up and move around for at least 90 seconds every 30 minutes. When you're at your kids' soccer practice, walk the sidelines or stand and watch instead of sitting. Don't take a chair!

- **The "lights out at 10:00 p.m." routine:** Get going on your sleep by 10:00. Try to avoid watching TV or checking your computer for 30 minutes before bedtime so that your brain is ready for sleep.

- **Get 8 hours of sleep:** Aim for 8 hours of shut-eye a night. If you get to bed by 10:00, this should be possible. It does you no good to stay up until midnight only to be exhausted throughout the next day.

- **The "plan to recover" ritual:** Every week, plan the day that you will recover from physical activity. Take it easy and let your body rest and repair. Don't skip this recovery day, as it's essential for keeping your energy up and your mind clear.

- **Sign up for at least one group event every calendar quarter:** a 5-K event, a 10-K event, or an organized hike or bike ride. This will expose you to many people who are living a healthy lifestyle and can help build your supportive social network.

- **Become an organizer!** Set up a walking group. When you're the organizer, you feel accountable to others to always make it happen.

MIND-SET AND POSITIVE OUTLOOK ROUTINES, RITUALS, AND TIPS

- **The "be grateful" ritual:** First thing in the morning, as you look in the mirror, take a moment to be grateful for everything you have. If the sun is out, open the curtains and take a deep breath . . . it's like a supercharger for your day.

- **Strive not to take everything so seriously:** The little things that get us down are usually unimportant in the big picture.

- **Cherish the moment:** Whenever something positive happens in your day or your life, pause and simply cherish the moment. Let the good feeling wash over you. Simply experience how it feels. The next time you feel blue, think about all the moments you've been able to cherish and how fortunate you really are.

- **The "go crazy when people aren't looking" routine:** Whenever you find yourself alone or with a trusted partner and no one else will notice, go crazy: Dance, sing, let it all out. Try this in an elevator sometime . . . we dare you not to laugh when the doors open.

- **Plan:** People who plan are much more successful at achieving their goals. Plan your meals, plan your shopping list, plan your physical activities, plan your recovery. The more specific your whats, whens, wheres, and hows, the more successful you will be.

- **Live in the present:** Focus on living in the moment. Don't think so much about the future. Develop awareness of when you are ruminating about the future and bring yourself back to the present moment. Enjoy the present.

- **The "healthy zoner" routine:** Take 3 minutes at least twice a day to do absolutely nothing. Focus on your breathing. Take in the world around you. Simply let your mind rest.

- **The "step out of your comfort zone" routine:** Once a month, try doing something that you would ordinarily not try. It may be taking a dance or yoga class, going rappelling, eating at a new ethnic restaurant, meeting up with people you barely know, or volunteering at the community center. New experiences are exhilarating, and you'll find that your confidence level will grow in everything you do.

- **The "lend a helping hand" ritual:** Giving of yourself to others can be one of the most gratifying experiences. Try volunteering at your child's school or at church or at a community event. Pick something active, like working for Habitat for Humanity. You'll recharge your happiness battery and make someone else feel good, too.

- **The "have a laugh" routine:** Look for humor in your day and in the world around you. Humor is great fuel for staying positive.

- **The "positive self-talk" routine:** Talk to yourself as if you were your closest advisor. Give yourself credit for the things you accomplish, even the little ones. A daily self–pep talk reinforces your goals and affirms your abilities to succeed.

- **Stay in touch with your purpose:** Always remember why you're pursuing your goal: What is the real reason that goal has value in your life? Remind yourself every day. Whenever you falter or feel tempted to quit, it's your purpose that will keep you going. Your purpose always trumps today's stumbling block.

- **The "hug a loved one" ritual:** Try cuddling/hugging with your kids, your husband, or your partner at least once a day. Focus on feeling the human connection and the synergy with your body's own rhythms. This is a great way to tap into the incredible energy that surrounds us all.

- **The journaling ritual:** Many people find that writing down their goals and their daily experiences helps them stay on track. It's a useful ritual to reinforce their purpose and also is an outlet for letting go of the stressors in life. They write about them to remove them from their daily thoughts . . . as if the stress were transferred to the journal.

INDEX